NARCOLEPSY

A FUNNY DISORDER
THAT'S NO LAUGHING MATTER

by Marguerite J. Utley

ORDER FROM:
M.J. Utley
P. O. Box 1923
DeSoto, TX 75123-1923

ISBN: 0-9643328-0-9 (paper)
ISBN: 0-9643328-1-7 (hardcover)
Printed in the United States of America
Library of Congress Catalog Number 95-90011

Cover design by author
Graphic arts by Jenny Hawkins
Printing arts by Darrel Eppler

ACKNOWLEDGMENTS

THERE WERE NO ghost writers for this book. There were many individuals who assisted with various aspects—from facts and ideas to proofreading and editing—at some stage of production.

I especially want to express my appreciation to the persons listed below for their contributions:

Sue Carella, Co-founder American Narcolepsy Asso., Co-founder Narcolepsy Network, Inc.

Meeta Goswami, M.P.H., Ph.D., Director, Narcolepsy Institute, Montifiore Medical Center, Bronx, NY

W.M. Jespersen, D.D.S. & Betty Jesperson, R.Ph., Duncanville, TX

Gila Lindsley, Ph.D., A.C.P., consultant, private practice, Lexington, MA

Edgar Lucas, Ph.D., A.C.P., Director, All Saints Sleep Disorders Diagnostic & Treatment Center, Ft. Worth, TX

Tell McDonald, Carlisle, PA

James G. Minard, Ph.D., UMDNJ: New Jersey Medical School, Newark, NJ

Ruth Justice Nebus, Co-founder, Vice President, Narcolepsy Network, Inc.

Glenn H. Nordehn, D.O., Duluth, MN

Charles P. Pollak, M.D., Dir., Div. of Sleep Medicine, Dept. of Neurology, Ohio State Univ., Columbus, OH

Niss Ryan, President, Narcolepsy Network, Inc.

Vernon Smith, Ph.D., Cedar Rapids, MI

Thomas G. Utley, Duncanville, TX

Pat Weaver, Amarillo, TX

DEDICATION

I DEDICATE THIS BOOK to my husband, CLYDE UTLEY, because...

Literally and figuratively, he has stood behind me to uplift me and uphold me in my struggles with narcolepsy.

He has accepted me as I am—whatever that might be at any given moment.

He has been understanding of me even when he could not really understand my problems.

He has treated me as a normal person yet made allowances for the fact that I am not normal.

He has laughed *with* me—not *at* me—using humor to turn weaknesses into strengths.

He has encouraged me in all my endeavors and worked with me to help achieve them.

He has been my proofreader, critic, advisor and greatest source of encouragement in writing this book.

Last, but not least, he has allowed me to sleep when I needed to and not made me feel guilty.

What more could I ask?

CONTENTS

PREFACE

PLEASE KEEP IN MIND there is no such thing as an "average narcoleptic." Narcolepsy is as distinctive as fingerprints and snowflakes — no two cases are exactly alike.

If you know a person with narcolepsy, the only thing you can rightfully *assume* is that he or she has a problem with excessive daytime sleepiness. That is the *only* symptom that must be present for a diagnosis of narcolepsy. If you are personally knowledgeable about a person's symptoms, then I hope this book will give you a better understanding.

On the other hand, if you know some excessively sleepy person, do not *assume* he/she has narcolepsy. Narcolepsy is only one of many causes of excessive daytime sleepiness.

Making assumptions regarding other symptoms or the effects of the disorder is an injustice to the individual. It may even do a great deal of harm. I would not want this information to be used to stigmatize or penalize the very people it is intended to help.

To My Fellow Narcoleptics

As you know, information about narcolepsy has been as scarce as hen's teeth. People who understand our disorder are almost as rare. I hope this book will provide answers to your questions and reassurance for you as a person with narcolepsy. There is nothing wrong with us — it must be the rest of the world. Seriously, we all need a pat on the back and a big hug. Remember, there are many others who share and bear the same burden.

This book is a long one for someone who has trouble staying awake. Keep coming back to it and you will eventually read your way through. I did.

TO FAMILY, FRIENDS AND SIGNIFICANT OTHERS

I hope that *seeing* and *hearing* the problems of narcolepsy from an "outsider" will give you a better understanding of the one "inside" your circle. Sometimes it is hardest to accept changes in those closest to us. If I could say one thing to you, it would be this: "*You* — not the medications — will make the biggest difference as to whether your friend or loved one is able to cope with narcolepsy successfully. It isn't always easy, but the rewards are great. My hat is off to you."

TO THE HEALTH PROFESSIONALS

I trust this information will help you to better diagnose and treat people with narcolepsy. But equally important, I hope it will help you to better treat the patient and not just the symptoms. You may have experiened excessive daytime sleepiness, hallucinations and even the equivalent of automatic behavior as the result of sleep deprivation — but not on a permanent basis that changed your whole life. Probably most of you have never witnessed a cataplectic attack. I hope that by sharing my experiences with you, I can give you a clearer insight into the strange world of narcolepsy and those who live there.

TO THE LITERARY CRITIC

While I have had a great deal of help from a good many people, I have not had an editor *per se*. I wanted to use my own style, which might not have escaped the cutting board of any self-respecting editor. It was important for me to say what I had to say in my own way. I could have had a *more* perfect book, but it wouldn't have reflected the real me.

INTRODUCTION

WHEN I SAY narcolepsy is a funny disorder, I don't mean that it is humorous. I mean it is a strange, odd, weird disorder. But to deny that its symptoms can sometimes result in hysterically laughable situations is akin to an ostrich sticking its head in the sand to keep from being seen. Since that trick obviously does not work, people with narcolepsy usually try to find more subtle ways to avoid the public eye.

Most disorders require coping skills, which the most successful overcomers use to advantage. I have found laughter to be one of my biggest allies as well as the biggest cause of my downfalls (cataplectic attacks causing loss of muscle control). Since some of my symptoms—or consequences thereof—are downright funny, I have found it is far better to laugh at myself and let others laugh *with* me than to let them laugh *at* me.

Laughter is good medicine. It reaches into the innermost parts of the soul that cannot be touched by drugs. It makes us resilient and gives us the strength to pick ourselves up, dust ourselves off and go on about our business. It helps us to maintain a healthy perspective about our problems.

While laughter is good medicine, tears are a healing balm. "There is a time for laughter and there is a time for tears" (Eccl. 3:4). There are times when I cry out of self-pity and frustration because of the limitations and restraints imposed on me by my symptoms. But my mother used to quote an old saying, "Laugh and the world laughs with you. Cry and you cry alone." It doesn't help to cry alone for long. It's so much better to laugh.

I invite you to laugh with me at my funny experiences with narcolepsy. But I would never try to minimize the seriousness of the disorder and its potentially devastating effects. Hopefully, I can help you to become aware of the suffering caused by narcolepsy without making you suffer from boredom in the process.

Maybe you have already been introduced to this sleep disorder by a couple of comic strip characters. Li'l Abner (now a senior citizen) was well known for sleep-testing mattresses in store windows. Peppermint Patty is the little girl in *Peanuts* who has trouble staying awake in school. We all laugh at these antics, but I want to take you behind the scenes where there are real people who must cope with the not-so-funny, real life problems of narcolepsy.

BASIC FACTS
ABOUT NARCOLEPSY

NARCOLEPSY IS:

☐ A sleep disorder characterized primarily by persistent and excessive daytime sleepiness (EDS), which is usually the first symptom to appear. Other symptoms may or may not develop over a period of years.

☐ Easily identifiable when cataplexy, a sudden loss of muscle control, is present in addition to EDS.

☐ A neurological, physical condition; not mental, psychological, or emotional. It is thought to be caused by an abnormality in the wake-sleep area of the brain.

☐ Frequently undiagnosed or misdiagnosed as fatigue, depression or some other form of mental illness.

☐ Typically experienced a decade or longer before it is diagnosed; after seeing an average of five or more physicians.

☐ Believed to be of genetic origin with initial onset triggered by environmental factors such as abrupt changes in wake/sleep schedule, illness, accident, drug abuse, hormonal changes or viral/bacterial agents. Relatives of a narcoleptic person are eight times more likely to have some disorder of excessive daytime sleepiness.

☐ Apt to begin in teens or early twenties but may begin at any age.

☐ Diagnosed by history of symptoms and sleep lab tests.

☐ Incurable once it sets in.

☐ Never fatal in itself, but symptoms may result in fatal accidents.

□ Usually manageable with drugs, changes in lifestyle, counseling and support from others.

□ Unpredictable. Varies greatly among individuals as to onset and progression, type and severity of symptoms and response to treatment. Individual symptoms may also differ from time-to-time or over a period of time, but the disorder generally is not considered to be progressive.

□ Potentially devastating in its effects on self-esteem, relationships, education, employment, health insurance, social life, activities, and quality of life in general.

□ Found equally in both sexes.

□ Affects an estimated 150,000–250,000 people in the U.S., most of whom have not been diagnosed.

□ Found in all races but not in equal proportions. Japan reports a much higher prevalence rate, Israel a much lower rate than that of the United States. Reasons for the reported differences are not yet known.

Symptoms of Narcolepsy

Excessive Daytime Sleepiness

Continuing susceptibility to falling asleep any time and anywhere on a fairly regular basis. Sleepiness may persist regardless of how much sleep a person has had. Sleep attacks can be uncontrollable.

Cataplexy (Cataplectic Attack)

Sudden, brief loss of muscle control, usually triggered by emotions such as laughter, anger, fear or surprise. Feeling of weakness, limp/twitching muscles or total body collapse. Inability to speak clearly if at all. Person remains conscious.

Hypnagogic Hallucinations

Vivid, realistic, often frightening dreams while going to sleep or waking up. They may include images, sound, touch and even smell.

Sleep Paralysis

Brief partial or total paralysis of the voluntary muscles when going to sleep or waking up.

Automatic Behavior

Familiar, routine or boring tasks are performed without full conscious awareness. Actions may not be recalled later.

DISRUPTED NIGHTTIME SLEEP

Quickly falling asleep may be followed by several/many arousals during the night for various reasons, including disturbing dreams. May be followed by fatigue the next morning, but is not a *cause* of EDS.

SLEEP DISORDERS

SLEEP RESEARCHERS have identified approximately one hundred sleep disorders and classified them as follows:

☐ *Intrinsic:* Sleep disorders caused by internal abnormalities. These include: narcolepsy, sleep apnea, periodic limb movements of sleep (PLMS) and some types of insomnia.

☐ *Extrinsic:* Sleep disorders caused by external conditions. These disorders can usually be resolved if the causative factor is removed. They include poor sleeping habits and alcohol dependency.

☐ *Circadian:* Sleep disorders involving disturbances of the sleep-wake cycle or one's biological clock. These include shift work and jet lag.

☐ *Parasomnias:* Sleep disorders which occur during sleep but are not caused by abnormal sleep processes. These include sleepwalking, bedwetting and night terrors.

Narcolepsy and sleep apnea, two primary sleep disorders, frequently occur together. Another sleep disorder that occurs more rarely with narcolepsy is periodic limb movements of sleep (PLMS). In both of these disorders, specific sleep disturbances cause multiple arousals during the night, resulting in excessive sleepiness the next day. If these disorders exist in addition to narcolepsy, it is critical that they be identified through an overnight sleep study. All underlying causes of EDS must be treated in order to provide effective management of symptoms.

SLEEP APNEA

There are two types of sleep apnea:

☐ *Obstructive sleep apnea* occurs when the airway collapses during sleep. This collapse results in cessation of airflow for several seconds. During this time, oxygen levels drop and breathing becomes more vigorous, forcing the airway open. The resumption of breathing may be accompanied by a loud snort and jerking of the arms, legs or whole body. After this momentary arousal, the person goes back to sleep and the process is repeated over and over again—perhaps several hundred times during the night. Loud snoring is usually a problem for the affected person and anyone within hearing range.

☐ *Central sleep apnea*, which is less common, occurs when the brain fails to send a signal to the chest and diaphragm to keep breathing. When the signal does comes through, breathing is quietly resumed without the snort and jerks associated with obstructive apnea.

Sleep apnea is a very serious and potentially life-threatening condition. The episodes of apnea during sleep can cause various organ systems to function abnormally and possibly contribute to hypertension, high blood pressure and a stroke. The use of certain drugs such as alcohol, sleeping pills, tranquilizers and barbiturates can be fatal in sleep apnea patients. The disorder is most prevalent in overweight, middle-age males.

Sleep apnea is diagnosed by an overnight sleep study at a sleep disorders center. Treatment varies, but techniques include: improving sleep hygiene, losing weight, use of a breathing machine (CPAP: Continuous Positive Airway Pressure), oral appliances and surgery. For information contact:
American Sleep Apnea Association
P.O. Box 66
Belmont, MA 02178
617/489-4441; Fax 617/489-4761

PERIODIC LIMB MOVEMENTS OF SLEEP (PLMS)

PLMS are usually experienced as leg jerks involving extension of the big toe and partial flexion or extension of the ankle, knee and hip. Each movement lasts up to 5 seconds and contractions occur at regular intervals of 10–120 seconds. Episodes are reported most frequently during the first part of the night, with the best sleep coming in the early morning hours. Although the person may be unaware of these movements, they cause multiple arousals during the night. The consequence of this disrupted sleep may be excessive daytime sleepiness the next day.

Treatment includes avoidance of anything that makes the problem worse, such as stimulant medications and caffeine; and the use of things to make the problem better, such as keeping the legs warm and a variety of medications. The disorder is diagnosed by an overnight sleep study.

People who have PLMS nearly always suffer from *restless legs syndrome* (RLS) during the day. This condition is often described as a "creepy, crawly" sensation in the leg muscles. Persons affected by this disorder usually are unable to keep their legs in any one position except for short periods of time before experiencing an irresistible urge to move them. The problem may become worse in the evening and make it difficult to fall asleep at night. For information contact:

Restless Legs Syndrome Foundation, Inc.
1904 Banbury Road
Raleigh, NC 27608
919/571-1599

SLEEP DEPRIVATION

W E RECOGNIZE the illnesses caused by cancer, heart problems, diabetes, AIDS, Alzheimer's Disease, etc. All of these are abnormalities. But sleep, which is normal and good, is having a great deal of trouble being seen as a threat to our well-being. Actually, it is not sleep—but the lack of it—that is taking on a villainous role.

Reports indicate that sleep deprivation in our country is nearing epidemic proportions. Our round-the-clock society has created this monster that is now out of control. Shiftwork, which is required to keep industry producing 24 hours a day, is partially responsible for the situation. So is the economy, which often requires people to hold down two or three jobs to make a living.

I see a large part of the sleep problem as a basic change of lifestyle in our society. In general, people these days are staying up later and getting less sleep—frequently from choice and not necessity. It is becoming an accepted way of life. Chronic fatigue is considered a status symbol.

Eight hours of sleep per 24-hour period has long been an accepted norm, with some people sleeping more and some less as individual needs vary. Eight hours was not an arbitrarily established time set by man. It was the amount of time people reported they needed to meet their needs.

Sleep *needs* for a population remain fairly constant over time; however, sleep *practices* do change. On the average, people still need eight hours of sleep—they just don't get it.

People who willfully ignore their sleep needs are in a state of denial. Their attitude toward sleep could almost be compared to that of an alcoholic toward alcohol. They will admit to not getting much sleep, as an alcoholic will admit to drinking.

But both groups refuse to admit their "habits" are a problem. Both profess to be in control of the situation, saying they can "handle it." No amount of talking to these people seems to have any effect. They will continue to "practice" until something, such as an accident, gets their attention.

While there are similarities in attitudes of denial, there is a huge difference in public knowledge about the two conditions. For years the public has been alerted to the perils of alcoholism, especially about drinking while driving. It is only recently, however, that information about sleep deprivation has begun to be disseminated to the public.

The U. S. Department of Transportation brings to our attention the fact that 200,000 auto accidents each year may be sleep related. Most of us are familiar with the incident of the oil tanker *Exxon Valdez*. This accident, which was one of the world's worst ecological disasters, was due to poor judgment by the third mate who had not slept in thirty-six hours. Shift workers—including doctors, nurses, firefighters and policemen—are not immune to the risks of sleep deprivation. And what affects them, affects us. We are all vulnerable—either directly or indirectly—to the hazards accompanying sleep loss.

When we use statistics, it is the numbers with the dollar signs in front of them that often speak the loudest. Much can be said about the number of accidents caused by sleepy people without creating much interest. But when the National Commission on Sleep Disorders estimated that sleep-related accidents in the United States cost at least $47 billion annually, that makes us sit up and take notice. It makes us want to ask who is paying the bill and what is being done to prevent this expenditure—if not the accidents.

Sometimes it is something more personal that finally gets our attention. Sometimes it hits closer to home when a truck driver falls asleep at the wheel and the 18-wheeler wipes out anything in its path. Yet there will always be those who say, "It couldn't happen to me." Don't be too sure....

CAUSES OF EXCESSIVE DAYTIME SLEEPINESS (EDS)

EXCESSIVE DAYTIME SLEEPINESS is not synonymous with narcolepsy. Although everyone who has narcolepsy has EDS, not everyone who has EDS has narcolepsy. Narcolepsy is only one of the many causes of EDS, which are listed below.

- Insufficient sleep/sleep deprivation (most common).
- Sleep apnea: commonly occurs along with narcolepsy.
- Narcolepsy.
- Circadian rhythm disturbance: biological clocks vs. imposed times; irregular sleep-wake schedule, jet lag.
- Use of drugs, including alcohol; withdrawal from stimulants, sedating medications.
- Psychiatric disorders/depression.
- Metabolic disorders: diabetes mellitus, first trimester of pregnancy.
- Periodic limb movements of sleep (PLMS): sometimes occurs along with narcolepsy.
- Neurological disorders: brain tumors, head injuries.
- Infections: "sleeping sickness," encephalitis.
- Miscellaneous conditions: "Long sleeping," idiopathic hypersomnia, and Kleine-Levin syndrome.

Do not confuse the disorder of narcolepsy with EDS.

1
EXCESSIVE DAYTIME SLEEPINESS (EDS)

EXCESSIVE DAYTIME SLEEPINESS is a complex, multifaceted condition. Only by looking at its individual components can you gain insight into this potentially disabling condition.

THE CONCEPT OF SLEEPINESS

Narcoleptic sleepiness includes the concepts of:

□ Drowsiness, sleep attacks and microsleeps.
□ Lack of alertness, dullness of mind and lethargy.
□ Fatigue and lack of energy.

These conditions paint an impressionistic picture of the sleepiness of narcolepsy. The image they create does not reflect a true likeness of the person but of the disorder. A distinct combination of symptoms and intensities blend together to make each case unique.

Drowsiness, Sleep Attacks and Microsleeps

Drowsiness

We tend to think of sleepiness as a brief, transitional stage bridging the states of wakefulness and sleep. People with narcolepsy also experience an unnatural "state of sleepiness" that may "come and go" throughout the day or "come and stay" for prolonged periods of time.

Sleepiness at night is a natural prelude to sleep. It is a welcome sign that sleep is on its way. Almost everyone is familiar with the feeling of irresistible sleepiness just before being overcome by sleep. It is that feeling of struggling to stay awake during those last moments of consciousness that plagues most people with narcolepsy on a daily basis. They may reach a peak of sleepiness several times during the day without the opportunity to find relief in sleep. Or they may stay sleepy continually. Sleep is not as welcome when it sets in at the wrong times.

Descriptions of the disorder frequently state that people with narcolepsy experience an *uncontrollable* need to sleep. It is true that some occurrences of periodic sleep episodes are uncontrollable, and sometimes sleep itself is totally overwhelming. But many people affected by this symptom will tell you that sometimes—under the right circum-stances—they can *resist* sleep or they can *fight* it off. But in passive situations from which there is no quick and easy exit (such as sitting in church, a meeting, or a concert), sleep is usually inescapable. In these situations, sleep is typically as sure and predictable as the tides.

On the other hand, if the person is in a position to get up and become active, the sleepiness *may* subside. The sleep episode may pass and alertness will be restored. Or that tactic may only postpone the inevitable. The person may continue to feel sleepy and will be more likely to fall asleep a little later on.

The fact is that sleepiness can occur any time and any place regardless of how much rest or sleep the person has had. No matter how motivated the person may be or how hard the person tries to stay awake, the need to sleep may take priority. These facts are key to understanding EDS.

A variety of things can happen while a person is in a state of sleepiness:

☐ The condition may continue for short or prolonged periods of time.

☐ After trying to resist sleep for some time, sleepiness may give way to automatic behavior, which is another symptom of narcolepsy.

☐ Sleepiness may give way to actual sleep. If dreaming begins, what the person is hearing may become incorporated into the dream.

☐ The person may hear, see or do something that will cause him/her to snap out of the state immediately.

Sleep Attacks

Typically, a sleep attack is distinguished from sleepiness by its sudden onset and overwhelming intensity. It may be, however, that drowsiness gradually increases to a certain point, at which time the person drops off to sleep. Narcoleptics may become so accustomed to functioning at low levels of alertness that they are unaware of the increasing sleepiness. Regardless of the technical aspects, some people seem to have a brief awareness that an attack is approaching. Others seem to suddenly drop off to sleep without warning.

The sleep experienced in one of these attacks is usually light, and the person is easily awakened. Sleep will usually last only five or ten minutes but may continue as long as an hour. Dreaming often occurs even during very brief naps. This fact which distinguishes narcoleptic naps from "normal" naps has become one basis for diagnosing narcolepsy.

Microsleeps

A microsleep is a few seconds of sleep that is interjected into the waking state. The duration is so fleeting that it may go unnoticed. However, depending upon the circumstances, a microsleep may be embarrassing. For example, a person may emerge from a microsleep thinking or talking about another subject. A microsleep can also be dangerous if it occurs during hazardous activity.

Lack of Alertness, Dullness of Mind and Lethargy

Lack of mental alertness, short attention span and poor concentration are characteristics of a sleepy mind. The mind longs to submit to sleep but begrudgingly labors to continue functioning. Efficiency, including accuracy and speed, is lost in the compromise. Learning and retention are affected. A person who continues to function in this condition is vulnerable to making mistakes and causing accidents. But poor performance has nothing to do with innate intellectual ability, personal responsibility, ambition, interest or motivation. It has to do with narcolepsy.

Dullness of mind and confused thoughts further exacerbate the problems. Webster defines *dull* as "Not quick, as in thought; sluggish; lacking in perception, sensibility or responsiveness." This seems to be an accurate assessment of the condition as it exists in narcolepsy.

Lack of alertness and dullness of mind worsen as sleepiness increases. Talking on a superficial level may seem normal but thinking is difficult. A person with narcolepsy who is scheduled to speak, would do well to be first on the program. Time and passivity are enemies of the narcoleptic mind.

Lethargy is yet another key dimension of this unnatural state. This term conveys a feeling of apathy or indifference. It is this perception of lack of interest that often creates resentment and hostility on the part of others. A person who is absorbed in a battle against sleep often does not have the capacity to focus on other interests.

Fatigue and Lack of Energy

These symptoms are close to the top of the list of complaints compiled by people with narcolepsy. They go hand-in-hand with excessive daytime sleepiness. They are so much a part of the symptom that patients sometimes report fatigue and lack of energy rather than the sleepiness. Fatigue and lack of energy are consequences of disrupted nighttime sleep with multiple awakenings, interrupted sleep cycles, mis-timed REM sleep and not enough deep, restful sleep. The same pattern is repeated night-after-night and results in day-after-day of chronic fatigue. It is possible for the tired-ness to go unnoticed when it is masked by energizing stimulants prescribed for EDS.

The combination of persistent sleepiness and fatigue is a losing combination. It takes energy to fight off sleep. If that energy is lacking, there is no line of defense and sleep wins out. In this situation, it helps to have understanding family and friends to serve as allies.

These same symptoms might be indicative of stress, emotional problems, depression or other unrelated medical problems. Fatigue experienced with narcolepsy is not to be confused with chronic fatigue syndrome, which usually is not accompanied by EDS.

THE EFFECTS OF SLEEPINESS

The sleepiness of narcolepsy can become the dominant force that dictates all other aspects of a person's life. Just how much of a tyrant it is depends on the severity of the symptom. Sleepiness is a very real, ever-present *force* to be reckoned with.

Whatever plans a person with narcolepsy may make are ultimately subject to cancellation at the last minute by sleepiness. Plans for each event must be carefully weighed by the possibility of sleepiness. This poses several questions seldom considered by others: Should I go? How will I go? Who will go with me? Where will I sit? What if I need to leave early or feel trapped because I can't leave? What if I go and fall asleep? Is it worth all the effort, frustration and disappointment if my plans don't work out?

Everything starts to become too "iffy!" Plans that should be simple soon become too complicated, and it's easier to

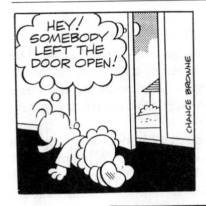

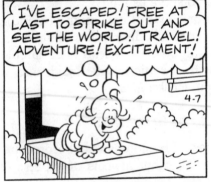

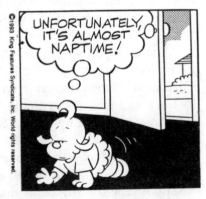

HI & LOIS reprinted by permission of King Features Syndicate.

"Whatever plans a person with narcolepsy may make are ultimately subject to cancellation at the last minute by sleepiness."

stay home. As more and more plans are ruled out, fewer and fewer ever come up for consideration.

Either consciously or unconsciously, many people with narcolepsy begin to wonder if it is worth the effort. Perhaps it is better, safer, more comfortable not to go.... Such concerns can beget a pattern of withdrawal and isolation. Thus, lives affected by narcolepsy can come to be controlled by sleepiness.

SEVERITY OF SYMPTOMS

Actually it is not appropriate to lump all people with narcolepsy together in one group. Some people have such mild cases that sleepiness is merely an inconvenience. The others whose lives are more drastically affected can be divided arbitrarily into two groups based on the severity of their sleepiness. (This grouping is based upon levels of sleepiness only and does not take into consideration the effects of cataplexy or other symptoms.)

Group I: These people are awake and alert enough most of the time to be able to carry on a normal life. Or perhaps it is only the appearance of a normal life. Many of those with narcolepsy try to hide their sleepiness and sometimes dysfunctional behavior even from those who are closest to them. Of course, such attempts at concealment only add to their burden. Group I people probably function well if they can stay physically active and/or mentally stimulated. They manage to go to work and take care of the necessities of life. Often they have little energy left over to enjoy life's little pleasures. The most pleasant thing they can think of is taking a nap! If they are taking a prescribed stimulant to help them stay awake, it is probably only moderately effective. In order to get by, they have been forced to change their lifestyle. In essence, this may mean they have given up many of their activities in favor of taking naps. Younger people, who naturally have more energy and motivation, may push

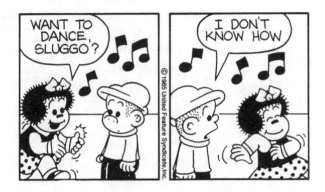

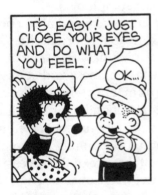
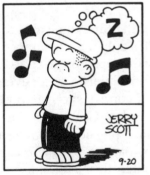

"The most pleasant thing they can think of is taking a nap."

themselves to keep up with their peers. But even for them it may be a struggle. This generalized picture of the life of a person with narcolepsy may seem bleak, but it is bright compared to that of the people in Group II.

It would be unfair to say that narcolepsy has little effect on this first group because their symptoms are mild. Even mild symptoms can cause serious problems. We must recognize, too, that certain factors can make a world of difference. What might seem like minor problems to one person may be devastating to another. Some people's circumstances allow for more flexibility, some are better able to cope than others, and some have a better support system than others.

Group II: These people have the most severe symptoms of narcolepsy. Many don't *get* sleepy — they *stay* sleepy! Life for them may become a matter of going through the motions. They are functioning at such low levels of alertness that all energies are absorbed in trying to stay awake long enough and to muster enough strength to take care of the necessities of life.

They are the truly dysfunctional ones. They can be so incapacitated by sleepiness that they often lose their families, their jobs, their ability to drive and to be independent. They can even lose their motivation to do anything to help themselves. Such drastic cases are the exception and not the rule.

Unless these people receive help from some outside source there is little hope things will ever improve for them. Drug therapy might help them to stay awake, but that is only part of the solution. Some of these people may have taken stimulants previously but, becoming disillusioned with the results or with their doctor, they have dropped out of the program. That is why a comprehensive management program (see "Management of Symptoms," pages 97–113) offers the best hope of providing them with a good quality of life on a lasting basis.

EXPECTATIONS OF SOCIETY

Sleep is both friend and foe. We must have a sufficient amount to survive and function properly, but too much sleep robs us of life itself. Either too much or too little sleep affects our quality of life. It's like food — we need the right kind and the right amount to meet our needs.

The optimum amount of sleep depends upon individual needs, which include one's biological clock, circumstances and preferences. Surveys indicate most people need seven to eight hours of sleep per twenty-four hour period. Daily quotas in excess of nine hours or less than five and a half are rare.

Regardless of how many hours we sleep, the basic expectation is for us to be able to stay awake the rest of the day. Normally, we are expected to be able to stay awake during an eight-hour work period as well as to take care of personal business and chores at home. We add to that our own agendas, which may include various forms of entertainment, socializing with friends and organizational activities.

The "List of Things to Do" is extended by job overtime, educational courses, sports and fitness programs, children's extra-curricular activities, etc., and the body soon begins to signal "OVERLOAD!!" Today's demands on our time and energy are more than enough to challenge even an efficiency expert.

Now onto this scene of beehive activity enters some poor soul who is different. This person not only dances to a different tune, but has to sit out many of the dances!

This individual may well be intelligent, ambitious and motivated to get ahead in the world. But there is another drive that will take precedent over all others — that is the urge to sleep.

How does this sleepy individual fit into the scheme of things? How does this person attempt to reconcile the gap between demand and performance? Usually with great difficulty and a lot of guilt.

Most people who suffer from excessive daytime sleepiness are probably riddled with guilt. They feel guilt from within and guilt from without. They feel guilty if they can't stay awake, and often they are made to feel even more guilty when they nap.

Napping is an area of discrimination that has gone largely unnoticed except by those who are the targets. People who *must* nap feel the barbs of prejudice. Those people who do not need to take naps and who do not like to take naps are frequently very intolerant of those who do. The implication seems to be that napping is a waste of time or, worse yet, a sign of laziness.

It would seem even the diehard antagonists could agree one nap a day would not be excessive, unless it were like some people's one meal a day—from morning till night. Now some experts are even supporting the idea that the body was designed for at least one afternoon nap a day. This is not news to many of us who, along with our friends south of the border, are strong advocates of the siesta.

Unfortunately, in our bustling American society, there is no provision for daytime sleep—either in the form of accommodations in the workplace or in an attitude of acceptance. Although companies are now mandated by law to make reasonable accommodations for individuals with disabilities, any major changes with respect to sleep disorders will probably be a long time in coming.

Many people with narcolepsy are self employed because they cannot adjust to others' rigid, arbitrary time schedules. Many other narcoleptics work night shifts. Whether this is a matter of preference or necessity, perhaps it is due to the fact that on-the-job drowsiness is more acceptable at night.

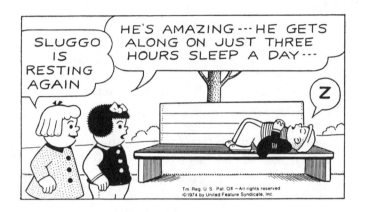

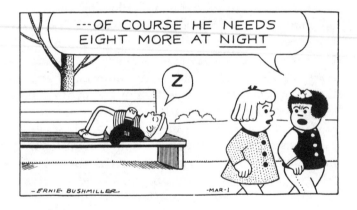

NANCY reprinted by permission of UFS, Inc.

People with narcolepsy and their families can relate to this cartoon — even though the idea is not supported by research findings. Studies indicate the total sleep time in a 24-hour period is not increased for narcoleptic subjects. Even though waking time may not be decreased, it is fragmented by the consistent, daily need to nap at short intervals.

Conclusion

People with narcolepsy cannot be judged by normal standards of conduct for sleep. For them, sleep does not behave in a normal manner—it misbehaves! This is a difficult concept for many people to comprehend and, consequently, to accept.

In ancient times, when people did not understand some natural (or unnatural) phenomenon, they made up a myth to explain it. Some people today do much the same thing. If they don't understand why someone can't stay awake, they may say that person is lazy or unmotivated or even stupid. Such assumptions are made of the same stuff as myths, that is, ignorance of the facts. And they must be combated in the same manner—with the truth.

Until the truth about narcolepsy is known and understood, those suffering from the disorder will pay a double penalty. Not only will they struggle with the symptoms, but they will be stigmatized as well.

My Experiences With EDS

BEFORE I RECEIVED a correct diagnosis of narcolepsy in August 1966, I had suffered the effects of this malady for approximately eight years. Being a "born sleepyhead," it was somewhat difficult to determine when "normal for me" became "abnormal."

By 1958, when I was twenty-four years old, the daytime sleepiness had become noticeably troublesome. At that time, I was working as an executive secretary in downtown Dallas. The *almost* over-powering urge to sleep beset me right after lunch on a regular basis. A lot of people get sleepy at that time. I just seemed to get a little sleepier. Sometimes it was possible for me to put my head down on my desk for a little "shut eye," which gave the needed relief. When my boss was out of town, I went into his office and had a good executive nap.

While the excessive drowsiness, as I prefer to call it, was frustrating and the struggle to stay awake was a hassle, it was not really threatening. But riding the bus home after work was a different matter. Fighting for a seat on a crowded unairconditioned bus in the middle of the summer was "the pits." (We didn't have that expression then, but it seems fitting now.) The ride home took about forty-five minutes. If I didn't get a seat immediately, I was able to sit down twenty minutes or so down the line.

The motion of any vehicle lulled me to sleep (the cradle effect), and the heavy exhaust fumes filling the bus added to the sedative effects. Within minutes of settling into a seat, my head would be nodding. I slept so much of the time that I didn't become familiar with the route. Consequently, since I couldn't wake up and tell where we were at any given moment, I had a constant fear of over-sleeping my stop. It never happened, but the threat was real.

Stress is frequently instrumental in the manifestation of narcolepsy. It does not cause the disorder, but it provides fertile soil from which dormant seeds may sprout. In retrospect, I feel sure the stress of marital problems was responsible for the onset of my symptoms of EDS at that time and the appearance of other symptoms at a later date.

A few years and many miles later (1963: Champaign–Urbana, Illinois), I was working at the University of Illinois Health Services as secretary to the assistant director. About 4:30 one afternoon, I had finished my work for the day and was desperately looking for some busy work to keep me awake. Cleaning my desktop seemed to be a worthwhile project that would "kill two birds with one stone." At the suggestion of another secretary, I obtained some ether from the clinic to do the job. I poured a little ether on a rag and, bending over my desk, started to work. It didn't take me long to realize I had made a poor choice of activities to keep me awake! The remaining few minutes of the day were spent in splashing cold water on my face.

Because of personal problems and/or drowsiness, I consulted one of the staff psychiatrists in his private practice. He placed me on Dexedrine, and I remained on that stimulant for the next three years.

Several landmark events in my EDS history happened during my two years in Illinois. I made a trip to Chicago and fell asleep while standing in line to register at the hotel. I didn't fall down, but I did actually fall asleep while standing on my feet. That night I went to sleep during a stage production of "The Sound of Music." A few months later, I fell asleep during a personal appearance of Helen Hayes! These were only the first of many performances through which I have dozed off-and-on and the reason I have virtually given up some of the more entertaining aspects of life.

In April 1963 my eleven-year marriage ended in divorce (due to problems unrelated to narcolepsy). "Free" to do whatever I wanted, I decided to complete my education at The University of Texas at Austin. It had been ten years since my first year of college and that was B.N. (Before Narcolepsy). Much had changed for the worse over the intervening years. To my dismay, I found I could not stay awake during classes!

The next three years could best be described as an ordeal. School had never been hard for me before, but this was a different ballgame. I felt as though I were starting out with two strikes against me.

Since I was on Dexedrine, I didn't sleep through all my classes. It just seemed that way. There's no way of determining how many extra hours it took because of my narcolepsy. It just took all I had. In addition to taking many extra hours trying to decipher my own notes, I had to borrow notes and work them into my own. I attended only the first two days of Chemistry classes—just long enough to find out the roll was not checked and the professor went by the book. All I had to do was study ten times harder than anyone else to make the grade.

I got a lot more than just "book learning" in college. I learned the fine art of deception, which is one of the chief coping skills of people with EDS. I don't mean the devious, low-down, lying kind of deception. I mean deceiving other people into thinking you're awake when you're not. The main trick is to be able to sit upright and keep your head from nodding. Even now, if my head snaps backward or forward abruptly, I very nonchalantly roll my head around a couple of times more to make it appear that I'm just exercising a stiff neck. Another trick to keep up appearances is to keep the pen in motion. Taking readable notes would be the real trick!

These skills still serve me well today. Maybe I haven't been fooling anyone except myself. If so, even that has served a purpose in helping me keep my self-esteem.

From the very beginning, I developed an "up front" policy—not of sitting up front but of being "up front" with my professors by telling them I had difficulty staying awake. I didn't want them to catch me napping and embarrass me in class. I had seen that happen before, and I didn't want to take any chances.

In addition to the "up front" policy, I adopted a "back seat" policy. That is, I sat toward the back or over far to one side in the most inconspicuous place I could find. I continue to practice these defenses. It's all part of a safety program practiced in one form or another by most people with excessive daytime sleepiness.

Just prior to graduation in August 1966, I was diagnosed as having narcolepsy and placed on Ritalin (details on pages 115-117).

Immediately after receiving my Bachelor of Science Degree in Elementary Education, I had a teaching job waiting for me in Houston. This leads into the problem of getting from Point A to Point B without falling asleep. Although it is not necessary for all those with narcolepsy, I virtually gave up driving on the highway by myself about 1961. When I reverted to single status, my mother assumed the role of chauffeur. She usually took the bus from her home in Pecos in far West Texas to our place of departure, a distance of 400-600 miles. Then after driving me to my destination, she returned home by bus. Life is not simple for narcoleptics or their families.

Out of such an experience came one of our favorite family sayings. I was really dreading the trip home one summer in the old car I bought to see me through college. The part I looked forward to the least was going down a very steep grade called Sheffield Hill in my old car with dubious brakes and pulling a trailer. I started worrying about that trip months in advance. Since I knew I would sleep most of the way, I cautioned Mother about the hill several times and told her to wake me when we arrived at the dropping-off place. True to her word, when we reached the spot, Mother announced, "Sheffield Hill." I sat bolt upright, looked over the situation and said, "Put 'er in second, Mother." Then I promptly went back to sleep. Now when we are prone to worry about things, my husband or I will simply say, "Put 'er in second!"

After a year in Houston, I found myself headed back to my home town of Pecos (home of the world's first rodeo and the world-famous Pecos cantaloupe). I stayed in Pecos for three years, living with my mother and teaching school.

Instead of joining the Baptist church in which I was raised, I decided to join the Presbyterian Church. I declared my intention to a member of the Board of Elders, who was also the superintendent of schools and my boss. I met with the Elders before Sunday morning service and satisfied their requirements for membership. As I understood the instructions, I was to go forward to join the church *after* the sermon.

I sat on the first or second row by myself (that is, without benefit of family or friends). After the first twenty minutes or so (plenty of time for me to have become addle-brained), I *thought* the pastor extended the invitation. Uncertain, but not knowing what else to do, I went forward. If I acted at the wrong time, the pastor was gracious enough not to embarrass me and the service proceeded in what seemed a normal way. Afterwards I was too mortified to ask. Sometimes it's better not to know....

One of the strangest phenomena I have experienced was having a microsleep (a split-second nap) in the middle of a sentence and changing topics in the process. My cousin's wife was driving me over to Tempe University out of Phoenix, where I was going to inquire about a master's degree program in English As a Second Language (ESL). I was talking to her about making application to Graduate School, when I stopped abruptly. Sensing I had said something wrong, I asked, "Did I change subjects—or something?" With a little prompting, I was able to recall I had started out talking about a college application and had switched over in mid-sentence to talking about an insurance application.

Instead of working on my master's degree, my interest in ESL led me in another direction. It was responsible for my receiving a fellowship with the Leadership Development Program, a Special Project of the Ford Foundation, for 1970–71. Unfortunately, because of my EDS and problems with drug therapy, I had to resign after only three months on the program. Massive doses of Desoxyn, Dalmane and Valium left me a "basket case." (See page 117)

I remarried in 1971 and at my husband's encouragement I went off all drugs. While my body took a rest from drugs for fourteen years, I managed to stay very busy in between naps. In 1975 we adopted an adult woman who was expecting her tenth child. (Her first four children were grown and she kept the baby.) We took custody of her five children (ages 4, 5, 6, 7 and 9) who were in a children's home. We thought we would have them about a year while their mother got back on her feet. However, things didn't work out quite that way, and we stayed in the parenting business for thirteen years. Since I was an only child with no children of my own, needless to say, this brought about some dramatic changes in my life!

At that young age, the children liked to take naps and just accepted napping as a way of life. They thought nothing of it when I had to stop in the middle of errands to take a short nap at the park. As a matter of fact, they loved it! They would play for ten or fifteen minutes and then when I honked the horn, they would come running. Their friends thought that was great.

Perhaps my biggest sense of guilt came from not being able to attend more of the activities in which they participated, but I simply could not stay awake. More than once I nearly fell off the bleachers. I was at almost as much risk of being injured as the players on the field!

In 1977 my mother became ill, and we moved her in with our already extended family. Although she was very forgetful, she always remembered I would sometimes get sleepy when driving. She never failed to keep an eye on me when I was behind the wheel and periodically she would say, "Now, honey, if you get sleepy, you let me drive."

For six years, I stayed home with Mother while my husband took the children to Sunday School and church. If I had someone to stay with Mother, I would sometimes meet the family for church. On at least two occasions that I can remember, I drove to the church, took a nap in the car and then drove home. I felt like the Lord gave me credit for trying.

Shortly after joining our present church, I invited the ladies to have their monthly covered-dish luncheon at our house. After lunch our new assistant minister rose to speak, and simultaneously my eyelids began to droop. I slipped quietly out of the room and headed to a back bedroom for a short nap. I set the timer for ten minutes, thinking that would be long enough—one minute to fall asleep and nine minutes to sleep. When I awoke, I noticed that the timer had already gone off. A glance at my watch revealed I had slept nearly an hour. Hurrying back to the living room, I found the extra chairs had been folded up, the kitchen had been cleaned, and the last guests were letting themselves out the front door. They even apologized for waking me.

An activity that most people find interesting and exciting sends me into a bout of depression within two days. You probably wouldn't guess—it's travel. Whenever I get in the car as a passenger, the first place I usually go is to sleep. This is often true on short trips (15–30 minutes) and virtually always true on longer trips (over 30 minutes). When we are traveling, my husband edits the scenery for me. Whenever he wants me to see something, he says loudly, "Look at this!" I sit up abruptly, look at whatever he points out, make a few appropriate comments, and then go back to sleep. Although

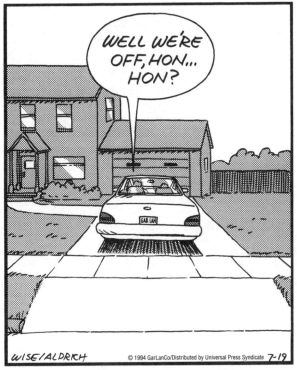

World's land-speed record for traveling companion falling asleep.

"Whenever I get in the car as a passenger, the first place I usually go is to sleep."

the drowsiness is not continuous, it begins to seem that way after several days of travel. It is so severe that I compare it to the feeling of trying to come out from under anesthesia — drifting in and out of consciousness. This is true even when I am taking stimulants. After a couple of days of travel and sleep, I begin to get depressed.

To end on a happy note, I'll confess I like to sleep. After I got over my childhood rebellion against nap-taking, I found that I really enjoy a good nap — especially after lunch every day. And that seems to be just what the doctor ordered.

2
CATAPLEXY

CATAPLEXY IS A sudden, brief loss of muscle control. Episodes, which are referred to as cataplectic attacks, are usually triggered by any kind of emotion: surprise, fear, anger, joy, sorrow and perhaps most frequently by humor — especially laughter when telling a joke. They can occur for no apparent reason.

Not all narcoleptics develop cataplexy, but there is no way to predict whether or not it will manifest itself at some time. Symptoms often begin several years after the onset of EDS. There appears to be a trend toward decreasing severity of cataplexy in later years, though this is not always the case.

Severity of attacks ranges from mild to severe based on intensity, duration and frequency. These elements of an attack vary greatly among individuals and even for the same individual from time-to-time or over a period of time. Fluctuations are thought to be caused by fatigue, stress, illness, hormonal changes, changes in medication or other, unknown causes. Abruptly discontinuing a medication may cause a rebound response that will increase all aspects of cataplexy (rebound cataplexy).

Intensity varies from a momentary weakness to total body collapse. A mild loss of muscle control may result in twitching or sagging facial muscles, drooping eyelids, a wobbly head, buckling knees, or the "giving way" of an arm. Perhaps the only evidence may be slurred or garbled speech due to affected vocal cords. Intense attacks can result in total body collapse and the inability to speak. When this happens, the

35

effect is much the same as when a puppeteer drops the strings to a puppet and it crumples to the stage. Until muscle tone begins to return, the person is virtually helpless and dependent on others.

Duration typically lasts from a few seconds to a few minutes. In rare cases, an attack may last as long as twenty or thirty minutes. Longer episodes can progress into REM (dream) sleep or distortions of reality such as that experienced during hypnagogic hallucinations.

Frequency varies from an occasional attack to many episodes a day. When attacks occur one after the other, it is called *status cataplecticus*. This rarely occurs except in cases of rebound cataplexy. When it does, it can usually be brought under control fairly rapidly by medications.

Cataplexy involves a partial or total paralysis of the voluntary muscles. Like other symptoms of narcolepsy, it appears to be caused by REM sleep (see pages 123–125) intruding abruptly into the waking state. The loss of muscle control during a cataplectic attack is similar to the sleep paralysis sometimes experienced while going to sleep and/or waking up. It is unclear whether or not they are caused by the same mechanism.

Cataplexy is almost unique to narcolepsy. It virtually does not exist except as a symptom of narcolepsy. When it does occur along with excessive daytime sleepiness (EDS), the diagnosis of narcolepsy is assured. In rare cases, cataplexy is the first symptom to develop and in isolated cases it can be the only symptom (idiopathic cataplexy). When cataplexy appears as the only symptom, *preceding* the development of EDS, it makes the diagnosis of narcolepsy extremely difficult.

Unlike epilepsy, during cataplectic attacks the individual is conscious (except as previously noted in prolonged attacks). However, the person may be completely helpless and unable to communicate. Cases have been reported of persons

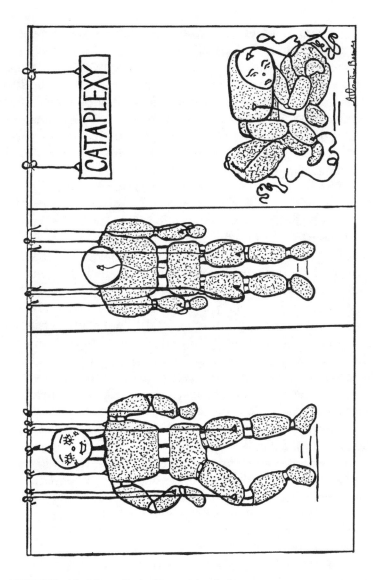

CATAPLEXY by Atlantis Brewer. Reprinted by permission of artist.

"...the effect is much the same as when a puppeteer drops the strings to a puppet and it crumples to the stage."

being taken to emergency rooms before recovering sufficiently to explain their condition.

Some people have no warning before an attack strikes.
With severe instantaneous cataplexy, the threat of bodily
harm is always present. If the attacks cannot be anticipated
or controlled, precautions should be taken by eliminating
foreseeable hazardous situations. Even then, the ever-present possibility of sudden collapse any time and anywhere
is a dangerous and discouraging prospect.

Some people have a warning sensation that gives them
a brief time to prepare for the attack. Perhaps they can sit
down quickly, lean against a wall or lean on a companion
for support. Much of the fear and embarrassment can be
avoided if there is someone who knows what to expect, what
to do, and who can speak for the affected person if necessary.
Unfortunately, this is not always possible.

Anyone who is subject to cataplectic attacks should
discuss the matter openly and freely with family, friends
and associates most likely to be present during an attack.
They should be informed about the disorder, what situations
are most likely to provoke an episode, what to expect when
an attack occurs, and what they can do to help. Think through
possible scenarios and decide on specific courses of action.
Everyone concerned will feel much more comfortable about
the situation if they are prepared in advance.

Individuals report very different preferences as to how
they want to be handled or more probably *not handled* during
these spells. Unless they need bodily support, many people
just want to be left alone and allowed to "come out of it" by
themselves. Others say "just a touch" helps. What works for
one may not work for another. But one thing you can be
sure of—they don't need sympathy. They need understanding.

If you have seen anything about narcolepsy on television,
it probably included research being done on animals. They
show cute dogs running around the yard and having a good

time. Then all of a sudden they collapse. You can almost hear the audience gasp and say, as with one breath, "Oh, aren't they cute! The poor little things!" It may look "cute" in dogs, but it is far less appealing when it occurs in humans.

A person experiencing a cataplectic attack is often the object of unfavorable attention (the center of a commotion might be more descriptive). Attacks are not only embarrassing but humiliating, degrading, mortifying and demoralizing. Consequently, those who are afflicted by this symptom struggle to find some way to deal with the problem.

Some people with cataplexy try to avoid these attacks by repressing the emotions that trigger them. When they feel the threat of an attack, they may try to mentally isolate themselves from their surroundings in order to maintain internal control regardless of external circumstances. They focus all their energies on remaining calm, cool and collected inside.

Instead of blocking out emotions, some people try to avoid situations most likely to elicit the emotions which typically trigger attacks. While this approach might help eliminate some attacks, it definitely eliminates many of the joys of life.

Repressing emotions and avoiding emotional situations may eventually lead to personality changes. For example, an outgoing person may adopt a reserved demeanor as a way of coping with cataplexy.

Some of those afflicted by cataplexy eventually come to the opinion that it is more advantageous to stay in a safe home environment whenever possible rather than run the risk of embarrassment. Sometimes staying home is a sentence rather than a choice and home becomes a place of confinement.

If attacks do occur and cause poor performance and/or embarrassment, it isn't long before there are repercussions of some sort. Whether it's on the job, in school, on the playing field, in social situations or wherever — the consequences can be devastating. At this point, we are not just talking about collapsing muscles, we're talking about the person's world collapsing. That would seem to put the problem in the proper perspective.

There are no happy solutions unless this symptom can be brought under satisfactory control, usually with tricyclic antidepressants. Cataplexy can usually be treated more successfully than EDS, but tragically many people are still undiagnosed and untreated.

MY EXPERIENCES WITH CATAPLEXY

MOST PEOPLE who experience cataplexy do so before they have a name for the condition. In all probability they have never heard of narcolepsy—much less any of the strange symptoms that comprise the syndrome. I was no exception.

My first occurrences of this symptom began in 1961. That was about three years *after* EDS had become quite noticeable and five years *before* I received a diagnosis of narcolepsy. Attacks did not occur on any regular basis until 1964 and did not become a serious problem for another three years. It was the summer of 1967 that lives on in my memory as *The Summer of Cataplexy.* (See pages 115–117)

I was living with my mother that summer and really needed her support, both moral and physical. Late one afternoon, as Mother and I were admiring the many nice plants in her back yard, we gazed up at the tops of her tall poplar trees. Mother suffered from vertigo and the upward glance brought on a sudden dizzy spell. The way she unceremoniously plopped down on the patio struck me as being funny, and I went into a full-fledged, total-body-collapse attack. Mother couldn't help me as she usually did, so I just sank down in a heap beside her. We started laughing and, still unable to stand, crawled up the back steps and into the house together! I'll have to admit that was one time the attack was worth the laugh.

When I start telling "war stories," my husband always wants me to tell his favorites. This next one is nearly everyone's favorite story. It happened in 1971 shortly after Clyde and I were married.

Two delivery men knocked at the door of our second floor apartment before bringing up the sofa I had sent to be reupholstered. As they returned to their truck for the sofa, my husband's sister said something funny. As my body started to slump, my husband caught me and laid me down on the floor—right across his feet. As I went down for the count, my full, short dress was pulled up to my waist, exposing my leopard-skin nylon bikinis. There I was on the floor, fully conscious of all that was going on but helpless to do anything about it.

In the process of trying to slip his feet out from under me, my husband pulled his feet out of his socks, leaving them under my prostrate body. My sister-in-law was standing over me saying, "My, those are the prettiest panties I've ever seen!" I was desperately trying to say, "Get me out of here," but my speech was so garbled they couldn't understand me. Seconds before the delivery men returned, my husband grabbed me under the arms from behind, dragged me into the bedroom and stretched me out on the bed. The first words I gasped were, "I thought I would die!" I meant that I thought I would die laughing. But my sister-in-law, who had never witnessed one of my episodes before, interpreted my words quite literally and was very concerned for my welfare.

Then, there was the time we went to visit Cousin Barbara soon after she moved to Dallas. Even as a child I always looked forward to visiting with my cousins, and I felt some of the old excitement. We didn't have long to wait as she answered our knock almost immediately. What to my wandering eyes should appear but Barbara in bright fuchsia booties standing on bright orange-colored shag carpet! Back in the days of yore, you just didn't mix those two colors, and the sight of that unlikely color scheme struck me as being ridiculously funny. Before I could even say hello, I knew I was in for a big cataplectic! My husband, who was getting used to playing catcher, caught me from behind, dragged me into the living room, and stretched me out on the floor.

This was the first time Barbara and her sons had seen such an exhibition, and everyone crowded around for a better look. Lying there—fully conscious but unable to speak—I found myself staring eyeball to foot at her fuchsia booties on the orange carpet. The harder I laughed, the more incapacitated I became. I knew I had to get "this thing" under control, but it took all the effort I could muster to regain my composure. As soon as I could talk, I tried to explain what happened, but that only sent me into more gales of laughter and another attack. Later we all had a good laugh. Thereafter, whenever we visited Cousin Barbara in the apartment with the orange carpet, I always had a cataplectic attack—whether or not she was wearing her fuchsia booties! (This effect is called conditioned cataplexy.)

A few years ago, we had a family reunion at our home in Dallas and afterwards some of us drove to West Texas to revisit the places of our youth. We had reservations to spend the night in Balmorhea, the picturesque little town at the foothills of the Davis Mountains, where I grew up. Leaving the others behind at the motel, I hurried down the familiar dirt street beside the little canal flowing through the center of town.

I was so full of nostalgia that I could scarcely contain myself. I almost felt like that little girl of bygone years. I passed the vacant lot where our grocery store stood before it burned down and saw the house my father built just around the corner. I paused just long enough for a wistful glance at my old climbing trees before hurrying on toward my destination.

I was on my way to see Lupe, our beloved maid who took care of me for eight years. I was doing fine until I knocked on her door, and then—Wham! My knees buckled, and I sank onto a stool beside the door. My head lolled forward, my arms fell limp at my sides, and it was all I could do to keep from falling off the stool. When Lupe came to the door, she didn't recognize me at first, and I couldn't tell her who I was or what was the matter. I had two problems of communication: my vocal cords were paralyzed and there was a language barrier. I couldn't speak Spanish and she couldn't speak English. We had always talked with our hands and a few broken words from each language.

She probably thought I was a crazy lady sitting there. I certainly must have looked it, and you couldn't have disproved it by me. We exchanged some rather puzzled looks before I was able to utter my first word, "Malo," which means "ill" in Spanish. It also means bad, and I didn't give any context clues. I could only hope she made the correct interpretation. But all was well that ended well. By the time the rest of the family arrived, Lupe and I were seated on her sofa, laughing and communicating in our own special way.

One of my big regrets has been that I have had to give up fishing. Like many narcoleptics, I can't stand up to the excitement. The instant I get a nibble, my arms go limp and I drop the rod. Actually, I haven't given up the hope of going fishing. I still carry a rod and reel in the trunk of my car. I've used it once in twenty-three years, so I figure I may get another chance. (Who says I'm not an optimist?)

I do not want to leave you with the impression that cataplexy is a laughing matter. So, last but not least, let me tell you about the only really frightening experience I've had. It happened several years ago, but the memory lingers on. I hope there are no repeats.

This cataplectic attack, like virtually all the others, was brought on by laughter. However, unlike other times, I dropped to my knees and my chin dropped down to my chest. In that position, my airflow was restricted and I began to panic. I was trying to cry out, "Help me!" but could not make myself understood. My husband was standing right beside me, but he was following the standard "M.O." (method of operation) of "hands off." Finally, he realized I was in real trouble and eased me back on the floor. After the attack subsided, I lay there awhile and cried quietly, as I often do with the really bad ones. I don't cry because I'm in pain or because I'm upset. It's more a release of tension.

I have been so much more fortunate than many people with cataplexy. During the thirty-plus years I have had the symptom, most of my attacks have been at home or at least within the confines of the family. My hands may shake and my knees knock while speaking in public, but I have never had a cataplectic attack in any situation where it really mattered. That is a lot to be thankful for.

My cataplexy now is very slight and infrequent. It isn't necessary for me to take medication to control it. When it does *display* itself, it is usually in the form of drooping eyelids, twitching facial muscles, wobbly head or weakness in my limbs. Typically, only one of these will occur at any given time, perhaps with garbled speech.

If I can manage to get my hand up to my face, I try to shield my face so it is not noticeable. If I'm sitting at a table, I try to put my elbow on the table and prop my chin on my hand. Of course, that won't work if my arm keeps collapsing. Actually, the whole episode is usually over in less than a minute and mostly goes unnoticed — except by my husband who keeps a keen eye on me!

Drugs that control or help to control cataplexy are life-savers for those who need them. That's a fact. But besides the physical danger, there's the emotional aspect of this debilitating symptom. The best treatment for this is understanding, supportive family and friends. I have the best.

Children, in their openness and naivete, are often the most accepting of our handicaps. Years ago, when our grandson Bryan was only ten, he greeted me with a big hug and kiss upon returning from a week of camp. Then he smiled and said, "I missed your funny face." ("Funny face" was his way of referring to my facial distortion during cataplectic attacks.)

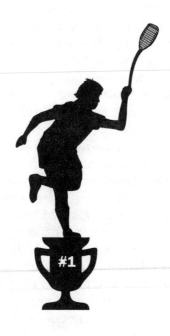

This trophy is awarded to
MARGUERITE UTLEY
for her success in mastering the fine art of
FLYSWATTING

For years, every time I started to swat a fly, my knees buckled and my arm fell limp and useless at my side—the flyswatter dangling on the floor. Refusing to admit defeat, I continued to go through my pathetic routine. After years of frustrated attempts, my unstinting dedication began to pay off. As my cataplexy began to improve, so did my prowess with the flyswatter. I found, much to my happy amusement, that I could measure my physical improvement by my ability to handle the flyswatter. Now, for the most part, I have emerged the victor over cataplexy and the lowly fly.

3

HYPNAGOGIC HALLUCINATIONS AND SLEEP PARALYSIS

HYPNAGOGIC HALLUCINATIONS and sleep paralysis are two distinct symptoms. However, they are so closely associated it would be difficult for me to discuss them separately.

Hypnagogic hallucinations are very vivid, realistic dreams that may occur when drifting off to sleep or awakening. They may take the form of images, sensations or experiences and may involve the senses of sight and/or sound and sometimes touch and smell. These dreams are frequently very frightening, especially when combined with sleep paralysis. Some people say they may also be wish-fulfilling or amusing. They are so life-like it is often difficult to distinguish them from reality.

These hallucinations seem so real because they occur while the brain is partially awake in the process of going to sleep; or partially asleep in the process of waking up. In either case, the brain is caught in a sort of twilight zone between sleep and wakefulness.

Normal sleep progresses through four stages of sleep, taking an average of about ninety minutes, before REM (rapid eye movement) sleep begins. This is the dream stage. Narcoleptic sleep can enter this stage immediately. When dreaming begins before the brain is fully asleep, fantasies seem to come to life.

These hallucinations are the weirdest of the weird symptoms associated with narcolepsy. They are what make some people with narcolepsy think they are crazy (and later sigh with relief when they find out they aren't!).

Sleep paralysis is a common, normal phenomenon that occurs during REM sleep. Typically, this partial or total paralysis of the voluntary muscles occurs while people are sound asleep and unaware of its presence. Because people with narcolepsy can enter REM sleep immediately, the brain may still be sufficiently awake for them to be aware of the paralysis. For example, an individual may dream he is being threatened and, at the same time, realize he is powerless to raise a finger in self defense.

Keep in mind these hallucinatory dreams are so vivid and realistic it is as though the person were living through the experience. Just imagine how you would feel if a knife-wielding intruder broke into your home and stood over your bed. Imagine the rush of adrenalin...the wild beating of your heart...the suspense...the screams....! Or worse—trying to scream or run and finding yourself unable to do so!

Think of the emotional trauma of one such experience. Something like that usually wouldn't happen to an individual more than once in a lifetime. Then think of going through similar experiences over-and-over again! If you can imagine that, then you might have some idea of how hypnagogic hallucinations and sleep paralysis can affect the lives of those who suffer from these symptoms.

When the same vivid scenarios recur time-after-time, perhaps over a period of many years, it may become difficult to sort out dreams from reality. Memories of dreams may begin to blend with memories of real life until it's hard to know which is which. If the distorted content of these recurring hallucinations is integrated into memory, it seems reasonable that counseling might be needed for imagined problems as well as real ones.

My Experiences With Hypnagogic Hallucinations and Sleep Paralysis

DURING MY INTERVIEW with the neurologist who diagnosed my condition, he asked about any experiences I might have had involving sounds during the night. I immediately remembered the chiming of the clock. It was the familiar, characteristic tone of the chime clock my father gave my mother for Christmas when I was about seven years old. I had counted the strikes many times over the years, but I didn't bother to count them that particular night. By the time I was awake enough to count, I knew that clock had been gone for many years. I loved the sound of the chimes when I was a child, but I grew to dread the haunting sound which continued to ring only in my imagination.

The doctor put a name to the symptom—hypnagogic hallucinations. Thus, the symptom was documented into my medical history as having begun in 1963.

During the next four years (three years of college in Austin and one of teaching in Houston), I don't recall terrifying experiences as much as I do humiliating ones. Several times a year I would make the twelve-hour bus trip home to Pecos to visit my mother. I usually went to sleep as the bus pulled out of the station in the evening and awoke when I arrived at my destination the next morning. I always had very bizarre dreams, and I suspected I said or did some strange things. Although no one ever said anything to me about any peculiar behavior, I thought they may have been too polite or too scared. I didn't ask.

Hearing voices (that aren't there) is another phenomenon frequently reported by people with narcolepsy. Some of my most memorable experiences in this area have come during daytime naps. I distinctly recognized the voices of family or friends as I listened to the warm, friendly flow of conversation coming from the next room. But as I began to wake up, I often realized some of the people I thought were there had been dead for many years. My memory recalled the sound of their voices as perfectly as though I were hearing the playback of a recording. Sometimes dreams of long-departed ones have been so real I feel as though I have been with them again. I consider that a plus—except that it makes me miss them more. Sometimes I wake up crying, more from nostalgia than sadness.

Because some of the experiences associated with hypnagogic hallucinations seem so crazy, individuals often keep them to themselves for fear of being thought insane. I have shared some of my most bizarre hallucinations with others of like affliction, but I have not "gone public" or in more contemporary jargon, "come out of the closet" before. Now in the interest of science and public education, I will "tell all." I may rename this *The Exposé of a Narcoleptic*.

Sometimes during the night when I am "asleep" in bed, I am absolutely convinced I hear a radio program. It may be a live newscast or it may be a wonderful symphony. Considering the fact I can't carry a tune, it is really a marvelous accomplishment to mentally reproduce the sound of a whole orchestra!

When this occurs now, I know—when I wake up—it was just a hallucination. But when I first experienced this happening twenty-five years ago, I was convinced that somehow my bed was wired for sound or I had a tooth that was acting as a receiver.

In the previous chapter, I mentioned that it is sometimes difficult to distinguish the content of recurring dreams from memories of real life. For example, I frequently dream that friends, whom I *believed* to be dead, are alive. In reality, these people have been dead for many years. The dreams themselves are not significant. It is what happens *after* the dreams that is puzzling. Afterwards I have trouble determining whether a person is actually dead or alive. Until recently, I thought the confusion takes place *after* I wake up. Now I have come to believe that it takes place in stage one sleep just *before* I wake up. When I am wide awake, I am—for the most part anyway—able to distinguish dream content from reality. This whole explanation may seem very confusing except to those who have similar experiences.

I seem to do a lot of thinking during the night and early morning hours, presumably while I am in stage one sleep. Some nights it seems to go on for hours. Thoughts must merge and mingle imperceptibly with dreams. Often the contents of these processes (whatever they are) are very creative and entertaining. But they are fleeting and elusive when I try to capture them upon awakening.

I have mentioned the weird and the bizarre, but I have yet to tell about the really terrifying dreams, which occurred during 1967–70 while I was living with my mother.

In the dark of the night and from my dream-like state, gray shapes would emerge and hover in the corners of my room. Phantom cats walked on my bed. I could sense the presence of evil in my room. One morning, after a particularly bad night, I remember saying, "Mother, I think there really are evil spirits that want to take over our bodies!"

These hallucinations were always accompanied by sleep paralysis that made it impossible for me to move. Even calling for help was almost more than I could manage. After several garbled attempts, I could finally call for Mother. My mother's ears, though growing old and hard of hearing, were still attuned to my cries for help. Roused from her sleep, Mother would hurry to my rescue. When she entered my room, the "things" in the shadows disappeared. Was it because her presence scared them away or because her presence brought me back to reality? Maybe it was some of both. I have since read that other people with narcolepsy sometimes experience psychic phenomena, including out-of-body experiences.

The vision of someone being in the room is a common one for people with narcolepsy. (I've heard from one person who actually called the police.) Many nights I have roused from my sleep with the feeling that someone is in the house — usually in our room. I get the same sort of feeling a dog must get when he first starts to growl and the hair bristles on his neck. I lie very still...not moving a muscle and scarcely daring to breathe...straining to hear any tell-tale sounds.... Lying there immobile, in a suspended state of fearful anticipation, I feign sleep. Long ago I decided that inaction was the safest course of action.

From the intruder nightmare emerged another similar one — or a projection of it. I dream someone is in the house, and I try to get up and check it out. But I can't move! Then slowly, slowly, I force myself to move — half-crawling out of bed and across the floor. I make my way to the light switch and flip it again and again without success. The light will not come on. In slow motion, I make the rounds of all the rooms, trying each switch in turn and finding none of them will work. I *know* the switches will work for someone else, but in my dreams I can never figure out why they won't work for me. (I can't even figure it out when I wake up!)

A variation on the theme is that I dream there are no light bulbs in any of the lamps or fixtures — which still leaves me in the dark! Maybe the dark is symbolic of sleep, and my failure to turn on the lights is symbolic of my failure to wake up. Who knows?

Sometimes I get my husband Clyde in on some of my "adventures." Recently I realized how really involved he was becoming when he related one of his dreams in which he told *me* to turn on the light. When I couldn't get the light to work, he tried to turn on the bed lamp — and it wouldn't work either. (Par for the course!)

One of our typical conversations might go something like this:

Me (in very low, whispered tones): "There's someone in the house."

Clyde (in sleepy mumble): "No, there's not—you're just dreaming."

Me (in a little louder, persistent tone): "There is someone in the house!"

Clyde (in a little louder mumble): "You're just dreaming—go back to sleep."

Me (louder, more persistent): "There's someone standing right there—don't you see him?"

Clyde turns on light, and in very firm voice, says, "*Now*, go back to sleep!"

One of the funniest episodes of this type went like this: One night I awoke with the feeling someone was in the house, and I kept trying to get Clyde to get up. Growing weary of my nudgings, he turned on the lamp. Sometimes I get mad (or so he says) if he won't get up. There was no doubt about it this night. I was *really* mad. If I had a gun and a burglar had been there, it would probably have been a draw as to which one I would have shot! I raised up on one arm, shot daggers at Clyde, and said in a very loud voice, "Spotlighting us when there's someone in the house! That's the dumbest thing I ever heard of!" Then I promptly went back to sleep.

When I woke up the next morning, I remembered the incident and my exact words. It's now another in our growing collection of family jokes. Once in a while—when it seems appropriate—one of us will say, "That's the dumbest thing I ever heard of!"

Recently we were returning home from a trip to Houston, when I asked Clyde if he heard me scream in the night. As usual, when we stay in a motel or hotel, I dreamed someone was breaking into our room. And, as usual, I let out a loud scream. At least I thought I did until Clyde said, "You weren't screaming. You were just dreaming you were screaming."

One of my favorite narcolepsy jokes is about a woman who tries to wake her husband when she thinks she hears someone downstairs. When he tries to tell her she is just having a bad dream, she asks, "Why is it every time I think I hear someone downstairs, you say I'm having a bad dream?" His reply: "Because we don't have a downstairs."

Strangely enough, I am trying to condition myself to recognize such discrepancies in my own dreams. For example, I often dream someone is coming in a window above our bed. If I can realize (while dreaming) that we don't have a window over our bed *now*, then maybe I can also realize it's only a dream. I understand from others that the technique really works.

A research study conducted by the Sleep Disorders Center at St. Louis University School of Medicine indicates that more than half of the spouses of problem sleepers fail to get a good night's sleep. If my husband were not a really sound sleeper, I'm sure I would keep him awake with all the talking and yelling that I do. I cannot emphasize strongly enough the importance of an understanding spouse.

I must confess I have not actively pursued treatment for these conditions. I have tried two antidepressants—each at a different time in my life—without success. But I did not go back to my doctor, tell him it wasn't working and ask to try another dosage or drug. Persistence is necessary for successful end results.

4
AUTOMATIC BEHAVIOR

THE TERM *automatic behavior* is very appropriate for this symptom. Webster defines automatic as "not voluntary; mechanical; performed without conscious intention." We all (even people without narcolepsy) lapse into this mode at certain times. Virtually any time we are engaged in performing tedious, routine tasks — especially over prolonged periods of time — we are prone to let our minds wander. This is true of production-line type work and jobs such as painting, ironing, and even driving.

Typically we refer to this mind-wandering activity as daydreaming. When a person with narcolepsy engages in this activity, it often *is* daydreaming. That is, it occurs during an episode of REM sleep that has intruded into the waking state. In one form or another, narcoleptics seem to spend a lot of time in which they are half awake and half asleep!

The body continues to function, going through the motions of performing familiar actions, even though the mind has partially retreated into sleep. The person may have little conscious awareness during performance of the activities and little or no recollection afterwards. Under the circumstances, it is not surprising many mistakes are made during these times.

A sleep attack that is ignored too long can easily turn into an episode of automatic behavior. Conversely, persons experiencing automatic behavior may suddenly drop off to sleep.

Depending upon the activity, automatic behavior can be potentially dangerous. Driving or operating hazardous machinery, activities requiring judgment calls, taking care of children; even cooking can be risky. Every person with narcolepsy needs to be aware of threatening situations and take precautions.

Misplacing things is a common occurrence during automatic behavior. High on the list of easily misplaced items are car keys, checks, letters, jewelry and other necessities. Anything smaller than a breadbox is fair game.

Occurrences of automatic behavior may be reminiscent of the proverbial absent-minded professor who was known to do all sorts of odd things. It is said the professor did such things as putting his umbrella to bed and standing behind the door all night. People with narcolepsy have been known to do such things as putting the dirty dishes in the refrigerator. A chef reported cracking eggs all over the kitchen floor, and a woman tells of putting ant powder instead of baking powder in the biscuits. Obviously, some mistakes don't matter and some do. It's of little consequence if you put the dishes in the wrong place. It's a lot more serious if you poison the food or put a decimal in the wrong place while doing your bookkeeping.

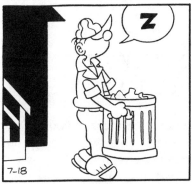

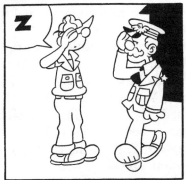

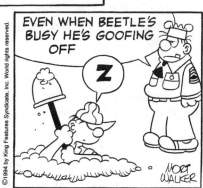

BEETLE BAILEY reprinted by permission of King Features Syndicate

"The body continues to function, going through the motions of performing familiar actions, even though the mind has partially retreated into sleep."

Unfortunately, many people with narcolepsy are stereotyped as "Beetle Baileys": lazy, dumb and indifferent.

My Experiences With Automatic Behavior

THE SYMPTOM OF automatic behavior appeared soon after EDS had become really troublesome. This was during the time I was working as an executive secretary. Taking naps when I could catch them helped me to cope with the drowsiness, but I was totally unprepared for the sudden appearance of the next disturbing symptom.

The day began in typical fashion and proceeded with business as usual until my boss called me into his office to take dictation. Even as I took the dictation, I was unaware anything was wrong. You will note the key word is *unaware*. As usual, I returned to my desk immediately and started reading over my notes before transcribing the letter. To my utter dismay, I had no recall of the contents. It was as if I were transcribing someone else's notes.

At that time, I had no idea the sleepiness and this phenomenon were both related to the puzzling disorder of narcolepsy.

About that time, I was driving back and forth between Dallas and Austin nearly every other weekend. Staying awake behind the wheel while on the highway had become a major concern. Even more disconcerting was the fact that I often failed to remember driving from one town to another. The weekend trips ended in about three months, and I don't recall this rather mystifying symptom creating much of a problem during the next few years. However, it had not disappeared but was lying in wait to torment me when I started back to college in 1963.

Taking notes, an act that is "automatic" to students, became a matter of "automatic behavior" to me. Almost invariably after a few minutes into any lecture, I entered the twilight zone. Part of my brain was on its way into sleep while another part struggled to perform its duties.

One particular incident in an English Literature class stands out in my memory. I thought I was doing exceptionally well staying awake until I glanced back over my notes. One word seemed to jump out at me. In the middle of a sentence, and completely out of context, I had written "erythrocytes" (red blood cells), which I was studying in Biology. That one word gave the clue that for a brief moment I had slipped into the land of nod (better known to me now as a microsleep). But, "the finger, having written, moved on...."

When I was teaching school, my "auto pilot" sometimes "kicked on" when showing a film or filmstrip. I went through all the right motions — start, narrate, ask questions, stop.... But when I finished, I wouldn't remember what it was about.

Another time my "auto pilot" took over for a few minutes in the middle of a lesson. I drew some geometric shapes on the blackboard and then stood back and looked at them in amazement. I don't remember what I planned to draw, but that wasn't it. I quickly corrected my mistake and proceeded with the lesson. I might add the shock of noticing such a blatant error is usually enough to snap me back to the state of alertness.

5
DISRUPTED NIGHTTIME SLEEP

ALTHOUGH THE PRIMARY symptom of narcolepsy is excessive daytime sleepiness, an erroneous assumption seems to be that sleepiness continues around the clock. As strange as it may seem, many people with narcolepsy find staying asleep all night to be as much of a problem as staying awake all day.

Dropping off to sleep at night is usually as easy as it is during the day. But this sleep may soon be interrupted. The remainder of the night may be filled with multiple awakenings and perhaps much tossing and turning.

The number of awakenings and the length of time it takes to go back to sleep varies among individuals. However, regardless of how many awakenings there were or whether they lasted minutes or hours, the overall feeling the next morning may be, "I was awake most of the night." These feelings may not be substantiated by nocturnal polysomnographic recordings. The perception seems to be largely attributable to numerous mini-arousals into light sleep as well as multiple awakenings.

The best quality of sleep is achieved when the stages of sleep within the sleep cycles progress in an orderly manner throughout the night without interruption. Unfortunately, there are some problems inherent in the disorder that interfere with the process. Abnormalities in narcoleptic sleep are responsible for mistiming of REM sleep, interrupted sleep cycles, more than normal amounts of light sleep and less than normal amounts of deep sleep.

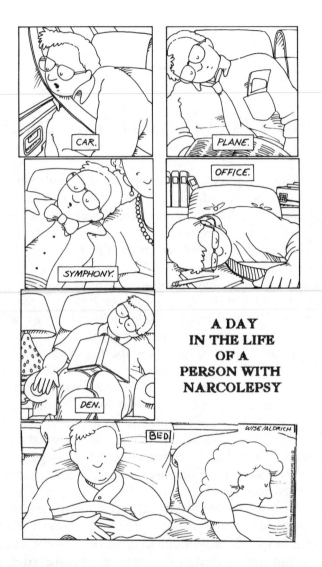

"Many people with narcolepsy find staying asleep all night to be as much of a problem as staying awake all day."

The problem with any condition or situation that causes multiple arousals or awakenings is they break the sleep cycle. As a result, the person misses out on some of the deep, restful sleep found in stages three and four. The loss of this restorative sleep causes much of the chronic fatigue that is a secondary symptom of narcolepsy.

In addition to narcolepsy, a person may have other sleep disorders, such as sleep apnea or periodic limb movements of sleep (PLMS). These disorders can cause hundreds of arousals that may not actually awaken the person but do disturb sleep.

There are numerous other causes for awakenings. Hypnagogic hallucinations may wake the person soon after falling asleep. If the dream is frightening or disturbing, or accompanied by sleep paralysis, the person may be glad to wake up to the real world. If the "ghosts" of the dream seem to linger and the feelings of fear persist, the person may be hesitant to go back to sleep for fear of repeating the same scenario. If it is necessary to become wide awake in order to shake off the vestiges of a nightmare, it may be difficult to get back to sleep.

Other sleep disturbances come from the carry-over effects of stimulants taken to combat daytime sleepiness, side effects of other medications, consumption of too much caffeine, too much sleep during the day or the need to relieve one's bladder. Stress, worry and illness can disturb anyone's sleep.

Doctors sometimes prescribe sleep-inducing drugs, but finding the right one for a patient can be a problem. Some drugs act to put the person to sleep quickly, which usually is not the problem with most narcoleptics. Other drugs are longer lasting and may have a carry-over effect the next day, compounding the sleepiness problem. Too large a dose can also cause this problem. If the person is taking antidepressants for cataplexy and/or other symptoms of narcolepsy, the problems of side effects and interactions of drugs are compounded.

My Experiences With Disrupted Nighttime Sleep

I CLASSIFY MYSELF as an insomniac narcoleptic (my own term), which means I am a person with narcolepsy who has trouble sleeping at night. I have a classic case of disrupted nighttime sleep.

It's as easy for me to fall asleep as it would be to fall off a log during a cataplectic attack. I don't sleep long at a time, but I usually go right back to sleep. (Some people aren't so fortunate.) My sleep is disturbed by bad dreams, and I often wake up the next morning feeling tired.

When I was on the stimulant Desoxyn, I would get up in the middle of the night and work for a couple of hours. I got a lot more done, but it wasn't a very healthful lifestyle. Somewhere along the way, I consciously reconditioned myself to staying in bed and going back to sleep. I still have to get up several times a week to shake off hallucinations. While I'm up, I check to see that all the doors are locked, get a snack and watch five or ten minutes of TV. By that time, I'm usually sleepy again and head back to bed.

Again I must confess to not putting forth a real effort to deal with this problem on a proper medical basis. After trying a couple of prescribed hypnotics that did not work for me, I gave up. I'm reasonably sure there is something that would be effective if I pursued the search. But like many others, I find that trying to regulate and deal with the side effects and interactions of several different types of medications is too much of a hassle.

Although I don't have much to say about my experiences with this symptom, suffice it to say that it is one of my biggest complaints! I really envy my husband's ability to sleep soundly and wake refreshed.

6
Other Symptoms

THE CLASSIC SYMPTOMS of narcolepsy, which comprise what is referred to as the narcolepsy tetrad, are EDS, cataplexy, hypnagogic hallucinations and sleep paralysis. Automatic behavior and disrupted nighttime sleep are sometimes referred to as auxiliary symptoms but often appear as part of the narcolepsy syndrome.

There are other, less specific symptoms which are sometimes associated with the disorder. These may be classified as secondary (the result of primary symptoms) or as side effects of drugs. Depending on how they are viewed, some of them may even be considered as consequences of narcolepsy.

CAUTION: The following symptoms may also occur as the result of sleep deprivation or other sleep disorders or conditions. These symptoms by themselves do not constitute narcolepsy but may occur as the result of it.

Learning Difficulties

Learning difficulties frequently present significant problems for people with narcolepsy. A sleepy mind that is not fully alert, difficulty in concentrating (especially for sustained periods of time), short attention span and confusion undoubtedly contribute to learning difficulties. This is predictable since listening and reading, the two basic learning methods, are passive states that almost invariably result in EDS.

During lecture-type situations, narcoleptics may exert more energy in trying to stay awake than in learning. After awhile they may lapse into automatic behavior, in which state they simply go through the motions of taking notes, turning pages, etc. When reading, their eyes may rove over the written page without conscious thought or comprehension. They may *read* and *reread* the material several times without having any idea of what they have *read*. Not only is much time wasted in these activities, much more time is required to correct mistakes and to get the job done right.

Obviously, much information is missed in the first place. Just because the senses have been exposed to the information does not mean that the brain absorbed it. And information received during this time may not be comprehended. These are learning problems—not memory problems. You can't remember what you don't know!

MEMORY IMPAIRMENT

Memory problems may follow *after* learning takes place. Not much is actually known about how narcolepsy affects memory mechanisms, but those with narcolepsy are very much aware the problems exist. Whether or not fully documented, explained or understood, the reality of learning and memory problems is evidenced by the consequences upon virtually every aspect of their lives. Education, job performance, relationships, self-esteem; ability and dependability are all negatively affected. Attention needs to be given to developing special learning and memory skills to compensate for these problems.

DISTRACTIBILITY (or ADD-Like Symptoms)

Attention Deficit Disorder (ADD), once thought to be a childhood disorder which would be outgrown, is now known to affect adults also. People with narcolepsy often complain of many of the same problems as those suffering from ADD. One of the main difficulties seems to be sticking with any one project long enough to get the job done, without getting side-tracked onto half a dozen other pursuits in the process. Frustration mounts when there is no sense of accomplishment in a job well done. This haphazard lifestyle of starting things and not finishing them is enough to drive everyone concerned to distraction. In some respects the similarities between narcolepsy and ADD are quite striking. While some genetic links are being explored, to my knowledge no *direct* connection has been found between the two disorders.

Distractibility in narcolepsy may be partly a learned behavior. In narcolepsy, people may condition themselves to evasive pursuits in their efforts to stay awake. Short attention span, poor concentration, learning/memory difficulties, as well as side effects of drugs, all contribute to the problem.

OCULAR PROBLEMS

Various eye problems sometimes experienced by people with narcolepsy include difficulty with eye fatigue, focusing, blurred and double vision, and involuntary eye movements (flickering). Visual disturbances can affect reading, which subsequently affects learning and further contributes to memory problems. They can also interfere with occupational and recreational pursuits or any activity which requires visual concentration. This is especially true over prolonged periods of time. Side effects of some drugs can cause double vision and related problems.

BINGE EATING (Snack Attacks)

The urge to eat can be almost as irresistible as the urge to sleep. This is an all-too-common problem among people with narcolepsy. There are several possible explanations for this problem.

Depression is a possible consequence of narcolepsy, and some people eat when they are depressed. Food may be used as a replacement for some of the many things in life missed by people with narcolepsy. Eating is sometimes used (misused or abused) in a fruitless attempt to ward off drowsiness and to help maintain alertness. Many people with narcolepsy seem to crave chocolate—a fact that is offered without any attempt at explanation.

Although it does not account for the urge to eat, it is only fair to point out that the ability to resist the urge may be somewhat impaired in this disorder. Sleepiness and self control have an inverse relationship: the greater the sleepiness, the less the self control.

Consequential weight gain may also be due to an increase in appetite due to medications such as Tofranil, an antidepressant drug prescribed for cataplexy. Lethargy may make it difficult to get enough exercise to burn off excess calories. Whatever the cause, the effect is that it all adds up to a lot of overweight narcoleptics.

SEXUAL DYSFUNCTION

Problems of sexual dysfunction may result from severe sleepiness and/or depression and sexual arousal-induced cataplexy. Impotency problems may be related to the effects of drugs, primarily tricyclic antidepressants, and possibly the chronic use of amphetamines.

ALCOHOL SENSITIVITY

An increased sensitivity to alcohol may cause a reduced ability to cope with its effects.

7
SIDE EFFECTS OF DRUGS

SOME SIDE EFFECTS of stimulants are so common they can almost be listed as symptoms. Stress, pressure and anxiety can intensify these effects, which include:

☐ *Hyperactivity, nervousness, excessive restlessness:* These effects make it exceedingly difficult to relax and they enhance irritability. They may also be responsible for incessant chatter, which can get on other people's nerves.

☐ *Irritability, agitation, mood swings and personality changes:* These effects make a person very temperamental and hard to get along with. They may also cause many problems with interpersonal relationships.

☐ *Heart palpitations (tachycardia; pounding heart):* This unpleasant condition can be alarming. Reducing dosage of stimulant may help.

☐ *Insomnia:* Carry-over effects of stimulants can cause difficulty going to sleep or staying asleep. Reducing dosages or taking medication earlier in the day may help.

☐ *Appetite suppressant:* Some stimulants act as appetite suppressants; potential for developing anorexia. Binge eating may occur when effects wear off and hunger sets in.

8
CONSEQUENCES

A FTER READING ABOUT the primary and auxiliary symptoms, the secondary symptoms, and the possible side effects of drugs, you might be to the point of thinking, "What! there's more?!" Unfortunately, there's a lot more. It's hard to assess the damage caused by narcolepsy because most of it is unreported.

Narcolepsy is insidious! The disorder frequently develops gradually over the years, and the person accepts the limitations and changes in lifestyle in increments. Not that they are happy with the new lifestyle forced upon them, but they become resigned to the seemingly inevitable.

Although the following problems may be mentioned elsewhere, they need to be acknowledged and recognized as possible consequences of narcolepsy.

PSYCHOLOGICAL AND EMOTIONAL PROBLEMS

Some degree of psychological and emotional problems are bound to develop in most cases of narcolepsy due to the inherent nature of the disorder. (If the underlying causes creating these problems are not clearly spelled out in these writings, read carefully and you will find them written between the lines.) Any condition that affects a person's life in the way and to the extent that narcolepsy does, will undoubtedly leave its mark upon the heart and soul.

The typical approach of treating the physical with drugs addresses only part of the problem. Attention must be focused on treating the whole person. (See "Management of Symptoms," pages 97–113.)

SOCIAL WITHDRAWAL AND ISOLATION

Narcolepsy is essentially a private struggle between the individual and the disorder. While some symptoms are visible, the effects are internalized. Perhaps it is the same with any disease or illness that sets one apart from what is considered normal.

Narcolepsy, like blindness or deafness, tends to isolate people from society. Many factors contribute to this problem:

- ☐ They can't stay awake.
- ☐ They are too tired.
- ☐ They can't participate in certain activities due to cataplexy.
- ☐ They are embarrassed by their behavior(s).
- ☐ They may be unable to drive or lack transportation.
- ☐ They feel less acceptable due to poor self-esteem.

Quality of life, in large part, depends upon our contacts with other people. When you lose touch with people, to some extent you lose touch with life, love and the pursuit of happiness. However, the effect of severed associations depends a great deal upon the person's temperament. If the person is basically a "loner," social distance won't make as big a difference as it will to the person who is a "mixer." Family and close friends also make a tremendous difference. Even a few close relationships help a person experience a more satisfying life.

LOSS OF INDEPENDENCE

Independence is the treasured dream of young and old alike. The young long to be old enough to be independent. The old long to be healthy and financially able to stay independent. Being able to maintain a place of our own and drive a car enables or empowers us, in large part, to live a life of our own choosing – to come and go as we please. If you have had to take the car keys away from an elderly person or move one into a nursing home, you have witnessed the trauma of having to give up independence. Sometimes loss of independence comes before old age. Sometimes it comes with narcolepsy – regardless of age! The degree of dependence is roughly equivalent to the severity of the symptoms. This loss does not necessarily come quickly, but subtly pilfers away individual freedom one piece at a time with a restriction here and a limitation there. This erosion may take place over a period of many years.

DRIVING RESTRICTIONS

The driving issue demands its place as a consequence of narcolepsy, but it cannot be limited to a small paragraph under a subheading. The subject is mentioned under "Loss of Independence" above, as well as under "Legal Matters." It appears in my experiences with EDS and automatic behavior. When the partial or total inability to drive occurs, the effects are far reaching and devastating.

ECONOMIC REPERCUSSIONS

The most serious economic consequence, of course, would be loss of employment. Sometimes rather than loss of a job, people with narcolepsy may be denied promotions or may even receive demotions if they are perceived as lazy, unmotivated, disinterested or incapable of performing the job satisfactorily. Sleepiness, cataplexy, and visual and memory problems are possible contributors to job-related problems.

Financial problems follow job loss or inability to advance on the job. Sometimes this has meant the loss of homes, cars and other property. Inability to get insurance coverage or having to pay a higher rate also has an impact on finances.

EDUCATION

Problems with getting an education develop with the onset of excessive daytime sleepiness. This may be in elementary school, college or beyond to continuing education classes. Success depends on the help received and the determination of the individual. In any event, the road will be harder, and the number who ultimately achieve their potential probably will be less. It is encouraging to note that there is evidence that people with narcolepsy are generally above average in intelligence.

FAILURE AND LOWERED SELF ESTEEM

The symptoms and consequences of narcolepsy work together to form a blueprint for failure and subsequent lowered self esteem if permitted to take its course. An early sense of self-worth and strong inner resources provide a firm foundation that helps to withstand the host of negative influences which can be present with narcolepsy. In addition, a comprehensive management program (pages 97–113) provides the best line of defense against these problems.

MY EXPERIENCES WITH
OTHER SYMPTOMS
AND CONSEQUENCES

AFTER MY FATHER died of Alzheimer's Disease when I was thirteen, my mother went back to college for five summers to get her degrees. She told me, "Honey, when I get through school, we'll live a normal life." I'm still waiting to live a normal life, but I'm not sure there is such a thing.

Over the years, it has become normal for me to jump from task to task. Not only do I have disrupted nighttime sleep but I also have disrupted daytime work habits. One of the biggest sources of frustration and dissatisfaction with myself comes from not finishing projects I start. For some reason this seems to be a common problem among people with narcolepsy—not all, but many of us. Typically, we are terrible procrastinators. "Mañana" is our theme song! We frequently lack self-discipline and can't make ourselves do certain things unless our lives are on the line—and even then we might hesitate.

Another plaguing problem is continual snacking—a more descriptive term for my habits than binge eating. Whether cause or effect, the outcome is the same.

One of my favorite snack foods is popcorn. I can always measure my degree of sleepiness by the amount of popcorn left in my chair and on the floor. The part of the brain that controls memory relating to where the mouth is located must be the first part to fall asleep. I think most of my popcorn-eating is done under the influence of automatic behavior. It also seems to me that the sleepier I get the more I snack.

So as not to leave out anything in this revealing exposé, I'll have to confess to irritability—as the side effects of stimulants, of course. My husband will tell you I have improved about 95% on Cylert (the stimulant I am currently taking) as compared to Ritalin or Desoxyn. I really was not a very easy person to live with. (Perhaps the fact that I don't have five kids and an invalid mother to take care of now accounts for some of the difference.)

When I remarried in 1971, I was under the influence of massive dosages of prescription drugs. But I couldn't have done better if I had been in my right mind. My husband has been the model supportive spouse. Apparently my narcolepsy endears me to him. He says if I die before he does, he is going to a narcolepsy group to find another wife! (With understanding, supportive husbands so difficult to find, I may be putting my life in danger by revealing this information.)

One of the reasons we have been suited to each other is that my husband is not the type who always needs to be "on the go." If he were, I don't think I would have been able to keep up the pace. I can't live life in the fast track.

Over on the side track are the remnants of my social life. Perhaps social withdrawal has made the biggest difference in my life. It has occurred gradually over the years, so I've grown accustomed to it. It's hard to say exactly what happened or when. Long ago I stopped meeting friends for lunch or dinner. Even if I'm taking stimulants, mealtimes are not my best times of day. The biggest obstacles to making *independent* plans of my own at any time are: (1) not knowing whether I will feel like going, and (2) never knowing for sure that I will be able to drive at the appointed time.

Whenever I am sitting still—in the movies, the theater, church, sports events, etc., *ad infinitum*—I may keep dropping off to sleep. The same is true if I am a guest in another home or the hostess in ours. Even if *others* don't have a problem with my somnolence, *I* do. Sometimes all of my energy has to be concentrated on trying to stay awake rather than on whatever is going on around me. When this happens, it is very difficult to carry on an intelligent conversation.

Even perfunctory responses such as clapping and laughing may be difficult to do at the appropriate time. This doesn't happen all the time but often enough that it sometimes seems that way.

The negative feelings associated with the struggle to stay awake begin to attach themselves to the desire to go or to the events themselves. Then I prefer to stay home rather than to struggle with all the negative feelings. Does that make sense to you?

Let me hasten to state that I don't believe this *always has* to be a consequence of narcolepsy. We may not always have to resign ourselves to being bench-sitters. In my case, things could have been—could be—different. If a social life were more important to me or to my husband, *both* of us could make more of an effort to improve the situation.

Narcolepsy does not bear the entire responsibility for my social withdrawal. Taking care of an invalid mother for seven years plus several moves to accommodate our changing family needs took their toll. Working at home rather than at a place of business has also added to the isolation. I have found it to be helpful to analyze situations and feelings in order to keep things in perspective. That way I am not so inclined to make narcolepsy the scapegoat for all my problems.

While I'm reminiscing, I think about the good old days before narcolepsy when I could read books. Maybe I will give it another try. If I could research information for this book, maybe I can get back into reading for enjoyment. Too often, I think, we give up because of discouragement and then become conditioned to doing without.

Analyzing my feelings in regard to being semi-dependent on others for transportation has led to some new insights. Through this experience, I have come to understand dependence as more than a physical inconvenience—it is also a mental attitude. Perhaps in addition to *being less able* to do things, it also made me *feel less capable* of doing them.

The impact of having to resign my fellowship program after three months because I couldn't drive on the highway was softened by remarriage two months later. I thought initially that I would go back into teaching but I never did. No regrets.

I would like to make it very clear that I never fell down—literally or figuratively—on any job. Instead of my work suffering due to sleepiness, I accomplished much more than I would have otherwise. I had to stay busy constantly so I wouldn't get sleepy. For example, I was never able to sit still at my desk long enough to grade papers while my students worked on an assignment. Instead, I walked the aisles giving individual help to students. People with narcolepsy can be better than average employees because they often have to put more effort into their work.

I've mentioned these sacrifices required by—or prompted by—narcolepsy because I think it is important for you to *see* the impact this disorder can have upon our personal lives. Some narcoleptics are not so severely affected; some much more so. The point is: some changes in lifestyle are almost always necessary.

One time I made the comment to my doctor that life is hard for narcoleptics. He replied, "Life is hard for everyone. It's just harder for people with narcolepsy."

In spite of my limitations, I have lived a busy, productive life and I am quite content. I have coped as best I could with these life experiences, but I wouldn't list all my methods as recommended coping skills. Perhaps the single greatest life-saving skill I have *learned* is *adaptability*. I had used the word *flexibility* until I asked my husband for his opinion. After what turned out to be a rather lengthy discussion, we agreed that I was more adaptable than flexible. Webster defines *adapt* as "to adjust to one's circumstances or environment." I think that is an accurate description of what I have done. I adapted to many different and unique situations, but I would have had considerable difficulty in adapting to punching a time clock.

9

DIAGNOSIS

STATISTICS INDICATE there has been an average of 10–15 years between the appearance of the first symptoms and receiving a correct diagnosis of narcolepsy. This lengthy delay is due to many factors.

One reason patients cannot receive a prompt, accurate diagnosis is that many doctors are not familiar with the disorder. Knowledge of sleep disorders medicine, which emerged around the middle 1960's, has been slow to permeate into the other fields of the medical profession. Until the study of sleep disorders is included in the curriculum of medical schools, as well as in continuing education courses, many patients will be misdiagnosed or undiagnosed and will go untreated.

Another barrier to seeking prompt medical attention comes from the way different people perceive their problems. Some sleepy people are in denial, refusing to accept and deal with their condition. Whether constantly complaining about being sleepy or suffering in silence, many fail to consider the problem worthy of medical attention.

Failure to report all symptoms to the doctor also makes diagnosis more difficult. Many patients overlook seemingly unrelated symptoms which, when put together like the pieces of a puzzle, clearly characterize the narcolepsy syndrome. For that reason, narcolepsy is often easier to diagnose from a case history after the disorder has progressed for several years.

In the case of children, the most frequent factor to delay accurate diagnosis appears to be that doctors do not consider narcolepsy as a possibility.

Narcolepsy is still in stage one of the problem-solving process, which is to recognize there is a problem. The situation will not change until both the medical profession and the public are informed about the disorder.

DIAGNOSTIC TESTS

Unless narcolepsy can be confirmed through a history of EDS plus the existence of cataplexy, the diagnostic approach should begin with an assessment of daytime sleepiness.

Evaluating EDS

In evaluating EDS, there are two objectives: (1) to confirm the existence of EDS, and (2) to identify the cause(s) of the EDS. This is a two-pronged process accomplished through clinical evaluation and laboratory investigation.

Clinical Evaluation

Clinical Evaluation of EDS seeks to:

☐ Differentiate between actual sleepiness and other symptoms such as fatigue and lethargy which may be misinterpreted as sleepiness.

☐ Distinguish between physiological (normal) and pathological (abnormal) sleep tendencies. It is normal for some people to require more sleep and to have a tendency to fall asleep during passive situations. The tendency to sleep is also influenced by environmental factors such as a warm room, a darkened room and the motion of a car. Abnormal sleepiness may be caused by other sleep disorders and/or conditions in addition to narcolepsy.

☐ Determine the presence of any other contributing factors such as: (1) stimulants (including caffeine and use of alcohol and other drugs) or withdrawal from stimulants;

sedating medications; (2) poor sleep habits including insufficient sleep or irregular wake-sleep schedules. (Sleep logs or diaries are helpful.)

☐ Determine age of onset. Symptoms beginning in the teens and early twenties are considered as positive indicators.

☐ Determine if other family members have/had EDS. Familial pattern is another positive indicator but not determinate.

☐ Verify sleep history by obtaining information from someone who has lived with the patient, preferably a bed partner. Observations by another party are often more detailed and accurate than what the patient reports.

☐ Assess the impact of EDS on the patient's life, especially in regard to family and social life, education, employment and driving ability.

☐ Measure sleepiness based on the patient's perceptions as determined by subjectively scored tests. The Epworth Sleepiness Scale is considered one of the most valid tests.

☐ Determine any medical problems which might affect EDS. This is generally based on a review of the patient's medical history rather than a physical examination.

☐ To determine if any mental or emotional problems may be present which might contribute to EDS. This information is based on psychological testing.

The clinical evaluation may confirm the existence of EDS but it cannot diagnose narcolepsy without the presence of cataplexy. Neither can it verify the presence of any other sleep disorders or conditions. This information can only be obtained by laboratory tests. Unless all underlying causes of EDS are identified and treated, excessive sleepiness cannot be effectively controlled.

A careful analysis of the clinical information should determine whether laboratory evaluation is required and, if so, what tests are indicated.

SLEEP TEST[*]

ARE YOU LIKELY to fall asleep while:

Passive State	Active State
Reading a book for pleasure?	Studying for a test?
Watching TV or a movie?	Playing table games?
Riding as a passenger?	Driving a car?
Sitting in a meeting?	Participating in a meeting?
Listening to a lecture or sermon?	Visiting with friends?
Sitting in a waiting room?	Eating a meal?

It may not be abnormal to get sleepy or to fall asleep sometimes during some activities, such as those listed on the left above. But if there is a pattern of falling asleep too often, in too many situations, it might indicate a sleep problem that needs attention.

If you get sleepy or fall asleep in more active situations, such as those listed on the right—except occasionally or for good cause—you might suspect a sleep problem. Good cause might include lack of sleep, being over-tired and side effects of medications, etc.

---

[*] This is not a scientific sleep test. It is intended for informational purposes—not a diagnostic tool.

THE EPWORTH SLEEPINESS SCALE[*]

HOW LIKELY ARE you to doze off or fall asleep in the following situations, in contrast to feeling just tired? This refers to your usual way of life in recent times. Even if you have not done some of these things recently, try to work out how they would have affected you. Use the following scale to choose the most appropriate number for each situation:

0 = Would never doze
1 = Slight chance of dozing
2 = Moderate chance of dozing
3 = High chance of dozing

Situation	Chance of Dozing
Sitting and Reading	_____
Watching TV	_____
Sitting, inactive in a public place (e.g. a theater or a meeting)	_____
As a passenger in a car for an hour without a break	_____
Lying down to rest in the afternoon when circumstances permit	_____
Sitting and talking to someone	_____
Sitting quietly after a lunch without alcohol	_____
In a car, while stopped for a few minutes in the traffic	_____
Total score:	_____

Scoring:
0-8 = normal, 9-12 = mild, 13-16 = moderate, 17-24 = severe

* *Sleep*, 14 (6): 540–545; 1991 ASDA and Sleep Research Society

Laboratory Evaluation

The following tests are usually performed in an accredited sleep disorders center by a registered polysomnographic technologist:

☐ *Nocturnal polysomnogram (PSG):* Electronic recordings made during an overnight sleep study. Tiny electrodes are attached to the patient to monitor brain waves, eye and muscle movements, and heart and breathing rates.

  The PSG alone is inconclusive in diagnosing narcolepsy because sleep onset REM periods (SOREMPS) occur in only 40–50% of narcolepsy patients and can be caused by other sleep problems. Results do reveal abnormalities suggestive of the disorder, which include frequent awakenings, sleep onset of less than ten minutes, and REM sleep onset of less than twenty minutes. The polysomnogram is especially beneficial in identifying other possible disorders of excessive daytime sleepiness, such as sleep apnea and periodic limb movements of sleep (PLMS), and measuring their severity.

☐ *Multiple Sleep Latency Test (MSLT):* A daytime sleep study designed to measure the patient's tendency to fall asleep. It is usually performed within three hours following a nocturnal PSG, while the patient is still hooked up to the electronic equipment. It consists of four or five 20-minute nap tests scheduled at two-hour intervals throughout the day. A diagnosis of narcolepsy is indicated if (1) the patient falls asleep within five minutes or less and (2) if REM sleep occurs within ten minutes of sleep onset in at least two of the naps. The diagnosis is virtually certain if other causes of early onset of REM sleep periods (SOREMPS) have been eliminated.

  Only about 50% of narcolepsy patients have REM sleep during the first MSLT. However, even if REM sleep is missing in the first test, a repeat MSLT will often show two or more SOREMPS.

The MSLT is the most widely accepted test for diagnosing narcolepsy as well as for grading the degree of sleepiness. However, it cannot identify the underlying causes of EDS.

☐ *Maintenance of Wakefulness Test (MWT):* A test designed to evaluate the patient's ability to stay awake. It is used to monitor the level of alertness and to grade the severity of EDS.

☐ *Electronic Pupillogram (EPG):* A technique designed to measure sleepiness by diameter of the pupil. Although the EPG is helpful in diagnosing sleepiness, there are problems that prevent it from being used as a diagnostic tool for narcolepsy. Another limitation of this method is that it cannot identify the underlying causes of EDS.

☐ *HLA (Human Leukocyte Antigen) Typing:* A genetic blood test which is generally performed only when a diagnosis of narcolepsy is uncertain. Research has identified a set of molecules (antigens) called HLA-DR2 and DQB1-0602, which appear on the white blood cells of about 95% of people with narcolepsy but are *not* present in about 20% of the U.S. population. A positive test showing the presence of these antigens is indicative of narcolepsy but cannot provide a definitive diagnosis. The test is most useful when it is negative, showing an absence of these antigens, because it almost certainly rules out the existence of narcolepsy. Most tests are for the DR2 gene only, but if the result of the DR2 test is negative, a test for DQB1-0602 should be done. A small percentage of persons with narcolepsy (especially African-Americans) are DQB1-0602 positive but do not have DR2.

Tests, especially the PSG and MSLT, are expensive, so it is wise to check with your insurance company in advance to see if they are covered. New lightweight equipment is now permitting ambulant home monitoring. Home tests, which are more convenient and less expensive, have a promising outlook for the future. Check with medical schools in your area to see if they provide sleep tests on a sliding scale basis. Free tests are offered periodically in connection with various research studies.

If your insurance will not pay, and you cannot afford the tests, the doctor must proceed by assessing your condition based on your history of sleepiness and all pertinent information available. (Remember, the presence of both EDS and cataplexy confirms a diagnosis of narcolepsy.)

FINDING A DOCTOR

Ordinarily you would expect a neurologist to diagnose and treat neurological disorders such as narcolepsy. In practice, sleep disorders are also treated by specialists in psychiatry, psychology, pulmonary medicine (for sleep apnea), pediatrics and other fields. In the early 1970's the ability to diagnose and treat sleep disorders came into existence and professionals from the various fields joined together to form the American Sleep Disorders Association (ASDA). This organization has developed accreditation programs for physicians, sleep disorder centers and laboratories, sleep researchers, and polysomnographic technologists.

Sleep disorders are best diagnosed at an accredited sleep disorders center where sleep lab facilities are available. It is usually preferable to get a referral from an individual who can personally recommend a doctor or facility. However, if you need help in locating a sleep specialist or sleep disorders center in your area, contact one of the sources listed on pages 157–158.

A knowledgeable physician can often diagnose narcolepsy by taking a careful history. However, this method cannot rule out the co-existence of other contributing disorders. Also there is an absence of information provided by sleep lab tests that is critical to optimal treatment.

A general practitioner or specialist in some other field may refer a patient to a diagnostic service center for testing. If narcolepsy is confirmed, and the referring physician does not treat narcolepsy, the patient may then be sent to a sleep disorders center for treatment. If the center wants to retest the patient in their own sleep lab, this can duplicate some costs as well as services. Advance knowledge of such practices can help patients to ask the right questions and make informed choices.

Any physician who has a patient with narcolepsy and who is not well acquainted with all aspects of the disorder should contact one of the sources listed on pages 157–158 for information. Some sleep disorders centers will share information.

Ask questions before making a first appointment. The information in this book will help you to determine whether the doctor is experienced and qualified in the field of narcolepsy.

- □ Is the doctor ASDA accredited?
- □ Do facilities include a sleep lab with a registered polysomnographic technologist (R.Psg.T.)? If not, where are patients sent for testing?
- □ What experience has the doctor had in diagnosing and treating narcolepsy, i.e., how many patients with narcolepsy has the doctor had?
- □ What are the fees for a first visit? Follow-up visits? Lab tests? Does the doctor give consultations by phone?

If you are not satisfied with the answers you receive by phone or with your introductory appointment, call someone else.

PREPARING YOUR CASE HISTORY

On your first appointment with any doctor, you are requested to give information about your medical history. If you are prepared in advance, it should help you to obtain an accurate diagnosis more rapidly. Perhaps just as important, it will help you to reevaluate your symptoms based on your present knowledge and understanding.

To prepare your own case history for narcolepsy, do the following:

☐ Make a copy of the "Checklist of Symptoms" that follows. Check the ones that pertain to you, making a note in the margin as to when the symptom began, how often it occurs, and other relative information.

☐ List any other doctors you have seen for this condition (with addresses and phone numbers) and dates you consulted them.

☐ List treatments for any symptoms identified with narcolepsy. Be specific, including the name of the drug, strength, dosage, how long you took it; its effectiveness and any side effects.

☐ List any and all current drugs you are taking and the condition for which you are taking them.

☐ List any other medical problems you have for which you are not taking medication.

☐ Be prepared to answer questions about your daily activities, such as: time you get up and go to bed, how much caffeine you drink and the number and length of daytime naps. Include information on the kind of exercise you get/take, including how much and when.

☐ Do a little medical genealogy research to determine if other members of your family have any disorders of EDS.

Your notes will not replace the verbal and written history solicited by the doctor, but they will help to get your case off to a good start in the right direction.

Checklist for Symptoms of Narcolepsy

Excessive Daytime Sleepiness (EDS)

__ You feel sleepy or fall asleep at inappropriate times and places, regardless of how much sleep you have had.

__ You experience sleepiness or sleep attacks on a continuing, daily basis—not just once in a while.

__ You almost always fall asleep during passive situations—watching TV, reading, waiting, etc.

__ You find it difficult or impossible to stay awake during some interesting and/or important events.

__ You are not as alert as you should be during the day; have difficulty concentrating.

__ You can usually fall asleep within 5–10 minutes.

__ You frequently feel tired and have little energy.

Cataplexy

__ You sometimes experience weakness in your limbs, head or neck, sagging facial muscles or garbled speech. These episodes seem to be brought on by emotions such as laughter, surprise or anger.

__ If you have experienced any of the above, you have been conscious and aware of what was happening.

Hypnagogic Hallucinations

__ You have very vivid (often frightening) dreams, see people or images, or hear sounds (especially voices) as you are going to sleep or waking up.

Sleep Paralysis

__ You have been aware you were unable to move or speak as you were going to sleep or waking up.

Automatic Behavior

__ You have done familiar, routine or boring jobs without being fully aware of your actions.

__ You have performed tasks and afterwards not remembered doing them.

Disrupted Nighttime Sleep

__ You wake up several/many times during the night.

__ You wake up in the mornings feeling tired.

Other Symptoms

__ You feel depressed — unhappy about your circumstances; unable to cope with your problems.

__ You have mood swings; feel irritable and grouchy.

__ You procrastinate; have trouble finishing tasks.

__ You have blurred or double vision; trouble focusing, eye flickering.

__ You are experiencing some memory problems.

Checklist for Consequences of Narcolepsy

__ You have trouble with relationships.

__ Your marriage/relationship has broken up.

__ You have given up part of your social life; various forms of entertainment.

__ You have given up personal pleasures, such as reading or handwork.

__ You have had difficulty in school; unable to continue your higher education.

__ You have been unable to participate in sports due to cataplexy.

__ You have been denied a job, lost a job, or had other job-related difficulties.

__ You have become unable to work and have filed a disability claim.

__ You have had to restrict or give up driving.

__ You have had an auto accident or other type of accident due to sleepiness or cataplexy.

__ You have been denied a driver's license.

__ You have been denied insurance, had exclusions for narcolepsy placed on your insurance, or been charged higher rates.

__ You feel bad about yourself (lowered self-esteem).

10
TREATMENT OF NARCOLEPSY

A LL DRUGS USED to treat narcolepsy are orphan drugs. They were developed for other purposes but have been found useful in treating the symptoms of narcolepsy. *No drugs have been developed specifically for this disorder.* Although a drug is not indicated for treating a certain condition, a doctor may prescribe any medication he believes to be in the best interest of the patient.

PHYSICIANS' APPROACH TO TREATMENT

There are two schools of thought among sleep disorders specialists in their approach to medications. The goal is not to cure the symptoms, since that is not presently a possibility. At best, symptoms can be controlled. The difference of opinion is over the extent to which symptoms should be brought under control, the maximum levels of drugs acceptable to do the job, and whether naps should be used to help maintain alertness and reduce the need for larger dosages.

Should the goal be: (1) to keep the patient awake and alert all day, regardless of the dosages needed and without benefit of naps, or (2) to keep the patient functioning at an acceptable level in order to perform daily tasks, using the minimum effective dosages and including therapeutic naps during the day to reduce sleepiness and increase alertness?

While the debate continues, currently *the most widely accepted approach is to prescribe minimum dosages and the scheduling of naps during the day.* The benefits of any drug must be carefully weighed against adverse side effects. Every drug carries with it a price to be paid in negative effects. The higher the dosage, the higher the price. It's better not to go into that kind of debt unless you have to.

DRUGS USED TO TREAT NARCOLEPSY

The following is a generalized guide to the most commonly used medications. Recommended dosages vary greatly. The current approach is to use lower dosages.

I. Central nervous system (CNS) stimulants used to treat excessive daytime sleepiness and automatic behavior:
   A. Methylphenidate (*Ritalin*): Sch. II stimulant: preferred drug. *Ritalin-SR* (sustained release) available. 10–60 mg/day.
   B. Amphetamines: Sch. II stimulants:
      (1) Dextroamphetamine (*Dexedrine*). 5–60 mg/day.
      (2) Methamphetamine (*Desoxyn*): not generally prescribed. 15–80 mg/day.
   C. Pemoline (*Cylert*): Sch. IV mild stimulant. 18.75–75 mg/day.

II. Stimulant used to treat EDS and cataplexy:
   Mazindol (*Sanorex*): Sch. III: less useful for severe narcolepsy. 4–8 mg/day in divided dosages.

III. Antidepressants used to treat cataplexy, hypnagogic hallucinations and sleep paralysis:
   A. Protriptyline (*Vivactil*): 10–40 mg/day. (Non-sedating; may improve EDS if associated with stimulant.)
   B. Imipramine (*Tofranil*): 25–200 mg/day.
   C. Desimpramine (*Norpramin*): 25–200 mg/day.
   D. Clomipramine (*Anafranil*): 25–200 mg/day.
   E. Fluoxetine (*Prozac*): 20–60 mg/day.

NOTE: With the exception of fluoxetine, all antidepressants listed are tricyclic antidepressants (TCAs). Most

TCAs have a sedating effect and should be taken at bedtime to avoid worsening EDS and stimulant interaction. (Some people find it necessary to take them during the day to control cataplexy.) Should not be stopped abruptly due to possibility of rebound cataplexy; should not be taken in combination with MAOIs (see below) or other antidepressants. May cause worsening of periodic limb movements of sleep and impotency problems.

WARNING: Prazosin, used to lower blood pressure, reportedly has produced dangerous side effects on narcoleptic patients using Ritalin and Vivactil.

IV. Monoamine Oxidase Inhibitors (MAOIs) (Not usually recommended due to potential hazardous reactions):
   A. Phenylzine (*Nardil*): May be useful in treating difficult cases of narcolepsy-cataplexy.
   B. Selegiline (*Eldepryl*): Has none of the tyramine-related side effects and may be useful in treating EDS.

V. Sedatives/hypnotics (to be taken at bedtime):
   A. Benzodiazepines (BZDs):
      1. Temazepam (*Restoril*): 15–30 mg
      2. Triazolam (*Halcion*): 0.125–0.25 mg
      3. Flurazepam (*Dalmane*): 15–30 mg (long lasting)
   B. Barbiturates: not usually prescribed.

WARNING: Should not be used if apnea is present. Do not take with alcohol; do not drive while under the influence of hypnotics.

NOTE: Information on drugs included here is intended only as a source of general information. Consult your doctor or pharmacist before taking any medications.

VI. Over-the-counter drugs:

Most nighttime sleep aids are antihistamines developed to treat allergies; can cause drowsiness as a side effect.

As with all drugs, product labels should be read carefully for directions and side effects. Check labels of pain, cold or allergy medications, which may have a stimulating or sedating effect.

New Drugs in Future

Modafinil, a stimulant somewhat milder than amphetamines, has been used successfully in Europe since 1986. It provides a more natural alertness for the control of EDS, but is less effective for cataplexy and other REM-related symptoms. It is undergoing clinical trials in the U.S. and should be available in this country in a few years. It may be especially useful in treating narcolepsy patients with heart disease and/or high blood pressure.

GHB (gamma hydroxybutyrate) is a natural substance used to treat cataplexy, especially severe cases. It is currently available in U.S. on an experimental basis only, but is being used successfully in Canada and France.

DIFFICULTIES WITH OBTAINING SCHEDULED DRUGS

Scheduled drugs are those tightly controlled by the U.S. Drug Enforcement Administration (DEA) and rated according to their potential for abuse and addiction. Schedule I drugs, such as cocaine and marijuana, were considered to have no therapeutic use. Schedule II, III and IV drugs are listed above.

Whether due to DEA efforts to control illicit use of these drugs or for other reasons, supplies of certain drugs are not always adequate to meet the needs of legitimate patients.

If you encounter a shortage of your medication, there are several possible solutions to the problem. Consider asking your doctor to prescribe the generic form of the drug, which is chemically the same. Because generics are made by different companies they may cost less and may not experience shortages at the same time. Having prescriptions partially filled or split among several pharmacies are other possible options. Although people with narcolepsy have legitimate needs, their attempts to purchase scheduled drugs are sometimes met with suspicion. Because physicians and pharmacists also come under close scrutiny by the DEA, they are sometimes reluctant to be involved with larger dosages.

Other obstacles to the availability of certain medications are raised by federal and state laws. Federal law prohibits automatically refilling Schedule II stimulants despite the fact that narcolepsy is a lifelong disorder. Some state laws prohibit mailing prescriptions for controlled substance medications and ban certain medications altogether.

DEA regulations restrict medications or dosages which they list as "indicated" for narcolepsy. If a drug does not appear on the list or the dosage is greater than the range specified, they are often rejected for insurance and Medicare benefits. In some cases, people cannot get their insurance to pay for the drug that works best for them and must accept one that is less effective.

Safeguards are needed to protect the rights of those who *must* take these drugs.

CARRYING CONTROLLED SUBSTANCES

In some states it is a criminal offense to carry a controlled substance (including your prescription medication) outside its original, labeled container. Even where it is not a felony, you run the risk of being detained by police if you are caught carrying any controlled substance in a pillbox, tissue, loose in your pocket or purse, in the car, etc.

Ask your pharmacist for a smaller container with a duplicate prescription label for convenience in carrying it with you.

11
MANAGEMENT OF SYMPTOMS

THE MANAGEMENT of the symptoms of narcolepsy should be a comprehensive program, including the following:

GOOD DOCTOR-PATIENT RELATIONSHIP

A good, working doctor-patient relationship is crucial to the effective management of symptoms. It must be a partnership, with doctor and patient combining their efforts toward the common goal.

Mutual respect is inherent in any good relationship. In impersonal relationships, it can be based on respect for a person's position rather than on character traits. The patient nearly always shows respect for the doctor's authoritarian position. It is equally important for the doctor to *show* respect for his patients.

A doctor's respect for his patient acknowledges that person's feelings, ideas and needs. It entails a commitment to treat the whole person and not just the symptoms. It involves good, two-way communication in which the patient feels comfortable in asking questions (with the expectation of receiving answers), expressing feelings and offering suggestions about treatment. It respects the patient's right to be involved in the process of setting goals and making decisions regarding treatment.

However unintentionally, the doctor often intimidates the patient. Frequently, the doctor doesn't have to *do* anything to cause this reaction. Many patients are simply intimidated by all doctors. Realizing that, doctors need to make a concerted effort to make each patient feel at ease. If the patient feels apprehensive, it slams the door on any effective communication. The doctor becomes the lecturer, with the patient a captive audience of one.

If the patient does not respect the doctor, perhaps another doctor should be consulted. If the doctor's manner or attitude causes emotional distress to the patient, there is little hope of arriving at effective drug therapy and management of symptoms. Under these circumstances, it is fairly certain that at some point in time the patient will drop out of treatment by that doctor.

GOOD COMMUNICATION SKILLS

Good communication skills need to be developed by all parties involved in the treatment and care of the patient. This includes doctor, patient and family. Frequently, the patient and family have little or no knowledge of these skills—which leaves the doctor as the sole source. If the doctor cannot assist the family in learning and applying these skills, then he should refer the patient to someone who can.

INFORMATION ABOUT NARCOLEPSY

Doctors must inform their narcolepsy patients of the basic facts about the disorder: symptoms, effects, consequences, possible causes and typical approach to treatment. They must also talk with their patients about genetic factors and the possibility that other members of their family may have the disorder. The patient should not leave the office without information on coping skills.

Physicians also need to provide their patients with literature they can take home. Regardless of how thoroughly the facts may have been presented, it is impossible for a patient to comprehend a verbal barrage of facts and be able to remember them later. It is a bewildering, frightening experience to be told you have such a weird disease, especially when the future is so uncertain. Being uninformed creates more fear. It is unconscionable to leave patients in a state of ignorance about a condition which has such impact on their lives!

Information about narcolepsy is hard to come by for the average person. With the exception of brochures, virtually everything that has been written is found in medical journals or reports available only within the medical profession. Unfortunately, the public is generally unaware of such educational materials provided by organizations and institutions. Doctors may order educational materials from sources listed on pages 157–158 or they may prepare their own literature. After the patient has had an opportunity to "digest" the information provided, the doctor needs to be available to answer questions.

REFERRAL TO A NARCOLEPSY SUPPORT GROUP

In addition to talking to the patient and handing out literature, the doctor *must* give a referral to a local narcolepsy support group if one is available. A support group is the link to others of like kind. Narcoleptics are the only ones who can truly identify with the problems of another narcoleptic. The importance of this cannot be understated. Referral should also be made to a national organization such as Narcolepsy Network, Inc.

DRUG THERAPY

Drug therapy is an essential component in the treatment of narcolepsy. Stimulants should help to relieve EDS and automatic behavior. Tricyclic medications usually help to control cataplexy, hypnagogic hallucinations and sleep paralysis. However, arriving at an effective drug treatment program for a specific individual can be lengthy and complex.

The process of finding the right drug or combination of drugs at the right dosages is not based on any scientific formula but on the trial-and-error method. The physician may start off by prescribing a stimulant for the control of EDS and, if required, a tricyclic antidepressant (TCA) for cataplexy. Treatment will probably begin with small dosages. If necessary, they will be gradually increased over a period of time until arriving at an effective level. Instead of prescribing higher than recommended dosages to achieve control of the symptoms, the doctor will generally switch to another drug in the hope it will work more effectively for the patient. Then the process is repeated for that drug. If the second drug does not provide satisfactory results, a third drug will be tried, or two may be combined. This "drug experimentation" may have to continue over an extended period of time. Therefore, patience, commitment and stick-to-itiveness are vital to successful end results.

Cases of EDS which fail to respond to recommended levels of stimulant medications should be reevaluated for other sleep disorders which may be contributing to the problem.

In addition to monitoring the effectiveness of the particular drug and the different dosage levels for that drug, the physician must also be on the alert for adverse side effects that might require changes.

Many factors influence the effectiveness of drugs, making it extremely difficult to arrive at optimal drug therapy. A drug that works well for one person may not work for another. One person requires only a small dosage of a drug to control symptoms while another takes a much larger amount. Some patients require treatment for sleepiness, cataplexy and other REM-related symptoms, as well as disrupted nighttime sleep. Each of these three groups of symptoms may require a different type of drug and drug interaction may be a problem. Even if a drug is effective, the side effects may be so bad a patient will opt to go untreated rather than endure them.

One thing that can be expected over a period of time is for the patient to develop a drug tolerance. After a while, the body may become accustomed to a specific drug or a certain dosage of a drug. Another possibility is that the severity of the symptom has increased and the drug is no longer controlling it. When this happens, the doctor has three choices: (1) increase the dosage of that drug, (2) put the patient on another drug, or (3) have the patient take a drug holiday and discontinue the use of that drug for a period of time. Rather than have the patient go off medication completely, the doctor may substitute another drug during the interim. When the patient resumes taking the initial drug, it may again be effective at the same dosage.

THERAPEUTIC NAPS

Too much sleep during the day is usually less of a problem than the amount of time usurped by sleepiness. While people with narcolepsy have little control over sleepiness intruding upon their waking hours, treatment does hold some hope in limiting its scope. The answer may lie in *therapeutic napping*.

Hours each day may be wasted in trying to fight off sleep. When the fog of sleepiness begins to roll in, the tendency is to struggle against it, stretching the sleep episode out over a much longer period of time. Sleep specialists are now recommending that people with narcolepsy schedule naps just *prior* to their sleepy times of day, which often occur about the same time. After waking refreshed from a 10–20 minute nap, most EDS-affected people can stay awake and alert for 2–4 hours before sleepiness recurs. Two or three 10–15 minute naps per day may be sufficient to get a person through the day in a highly functional state. Total nap time of 20–45 minutes — even an hour — could be very productive, especially in performance ratings. What an improvement that would be!

The scheduling of naps provides for a degree of dependability which is often lacking in the lives of people with narcolepsy. By counting on alert times following naps, the person can plan activities with more confidence.

Therapeutic napping probably will not replace the need for stimulants for most people. But supplemental naps possibly can reduce or help to eliminate inappropriate manifestations of abnormal sleep behavior as well as the need for larger dosages of stimulants. There appears to be nothing else available at this time that offers such substantial benefits.

My sister-in-law who had cancer always put a great deal of emphasis on "staying on top of her pain." If she could time her pain medication to take effect before the pain got too bad, she could keep the pain under control. If people with EDS can learn to nap *before* sleepiness sets in, they may be able to "stay on top of their sleep."

Therapeutic napping is considered to be an essential part of a comprehensive management program. As such, napping should be as acceptable for narcoleptics as insulin is for diabetics.

NOTE: People who do not have EDS, especially those who have not witnessed it in someone else, in all probability will not understand the concept of "scheduling" naps. They will wonder how you can possibly plan to take a nap at a time when you may not be sleepy. They will not understand—without some help—that those affected by this sleepy symptom have but to close their eyes and sleep will come.

HEALTHFUL LIFESTYLE

Illness, fatigue and stress can intensify all symptoms of narcolepsy. Knowing this, it stands to reason that the more people can do to reduce and prevent these factors in their lives, the better off they will be. (Isn't that true for everyone?)

Regular habits—especially in regard to sleep—are of particular benefit to people with sleep disorders. Getting up and going to bed at the same times every day helps to enforce individual circadian patterns governed by biological clocks. Some foods naturally have greater sleep-inducing effects than others. Timing and combinations of foods are also very important. Each individual should be alert to particular foods that seem to induce sleep or help to stimulate alertness and act accordingly. Anyone wishing to pursue the associations between food, mood and sleep should find abundant reading materials at the library or health food stores. (See also "Practical Practices," pages 135–136).

COPING SKILLS

Coping skills are as important to the management of narcolepsy as medication. Doctors must provide their patients with this information along with a prescription for drugs. Sending a patient home without this assistance would be like sending a one-legged man home with a prescription for pain—but failing to tell him he would benefit by the use of crutches, a wheelchair or an artificial limb. (See also "Practical Practices," pages 135–136).

COUNSELING

Narcolepsy is a physical, neurological disorder. It is not a mental illness. However, its symptoms sometimes produce psychological and emotional problems that require counseling.

Past studies of persons with narcolepsy often indicated they were opposed to counseling. This may have been because they refused to accept their problems as being of a psychological nature. But with changing times and attitudes, opposition is giving way to a greater acceptance of counseling. As people affected by narcolepsy become more informed about their condition and its consequences, they are beginning to seek help. These people want more than a "handout"

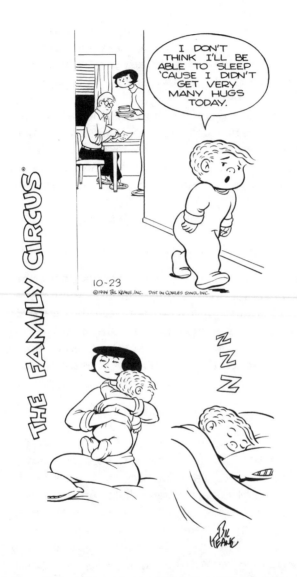

"Nothing has a more profound effect on a person with narcolepsy than the support provided by significant others..."

of a prescription for some drug. They want a management program that will help them adjust to the many lifestyle changes demanded by the constraints of narcolepsy.

Mental health experts tell us that when a significant loss takes place in our lives, we need to work through the grieving process. Persons with narcolepsy often suffer great losses in relationships, jobs, education, social life, ability to drive, etc. But how can they grieve, or who will console them when there is no recognition that a loss has occurred? These hurts are internalized and repressed rather than being recognized and treated.

Doctors must become more sensitive and responsive to the needs of their patients. They must treat the patient as well as the symptoms. These changes are long overdue.

PSYCHOSOCIAL SUPPORT

Nothing has a more profound effect on a person with narcolepsy than the support provided by significant others such as family, close friends and co-workers. Whether this effect is positive or negative depends upon the *understanding, acceptance* and *cooperation* of these people.

Much of the information that follows on the next few pages was taken from articles by Dr. Mark Flapan.

Understanding

Lack of understanding (or at least the perception of not being understood) is probably the greatest detriment to the well-being of any person with a chronic disorder. The person can better accept the illness than the fact or feeling that those closest to him do not understand. In this respect, we should all keep in mind the fact that it is difficult—if not impossible—to understand something you have not experienced.

Lack of understanding—whether real or perceived—is often equated with lack of caring and concern. This translates into hurt feelings which precipitate anger, which in turn tries to assess blame. Anger and blame evoke negative, defensive responses and matters go from bad to worse.

These explosive situations may be defused if all those concerned would learn to differentiate between hurt feelings and anger. Hurt feelings acknowledge some responsibility for the problem while anger blames the other person. If each party can admit some degree of fault, then there may be a willingness to work out the problems. Even the willingness of only one party can result in behavioral changes which will improve interpersonal relationships.

Many times family and friends do not really believe the person with narcolepsy has no control over being sleepy or falling asleep. They often think that if the person tried a little harder, really cared or showed a little more interest, he or she could stay awake. They think the person should be capable of doing all the things as B.N. (Before Narcolepsy). If others *knew the facts* about narcolepsy, they would know this is not so. If they had *understanding of the effects* of narcolepsy, they would not have such unrealistic expectations.

When others make unreasonable demands upon the person with narcolepsy, they set in motion another chain reaction. The person may be hurt and angry, but at the same time feel guilty because of failure to meet certain responsibilities — even though it is physically impossible to do so. Feelings of failure generate other feelings of unworthiness, self-doubt and lowered self-esteem. An intelligent, capable person may be as incapacitated by lack of self-confidence and poor self-esteem as by physical disabilities. On the other hand, self-confidence and good self-esteem, fostered by supportive family and friends, can help that person to be a successful overcomer.

Lack of understanding (or the perception thereof) is a two-way street. Not only does the person with narcolepsy feel misunderstood by others but that feeling is reciprocated. Others also feel they are not understood, their needs are not being met and they are not receiving the attention they require. These others may feel they are being treated inconsiderately and that unreasonable demands are being made upon them. There may be some validity to their claims. Family and friends do get neglected. They don't receive the attention and get their needs met as they did previously. But perhaps not for the reasons they perceive. Change has occurred as a consequence of an illness rather than because of some ulterior agenda. The person may no longer be physically able to meet responsibilities in the same way or to the same extent.

What started this endless chain of negative thoughts, actions and reactions? Was it lack of understanding or lack of concern and caring? No, most likely the confusion arose over attributing wrong meanings to what others said and did. It probably began with two culprits that go hand-in-hand: lack of knowledge and lack of communication.

How much better it would be to provide preventive measures rather than having to take corrective ones after the damage has been done. Many of these unhappy, unfortunate circumstances can be avoided if the diagnosing and/or treating physician sets up a management program for the patient instead of limiting treatment to drug therapy. (See pages 111–113)

Much misunderstanding can also be avoided if the physician will refer the patient to a local support group or even a national group which can provide information. A support group, better than any other source, can help the patient cope with the limitations and disabilities of narcolepsy. These groups offer immeasurable help to families — especially spouses — in coming to grips with the consequences of the disorder.

Acceptance

The person with a disability has a tremendous need to be accepted in "as is" condition. However, the person must first find self-acceptance before expecting acceptance from others.

Family and friends often have difficulty in accepting the fact this person is different from the person they used to know. They may be in a state of denial, refusing to acknowledge these differences exist and refusing to deal with the reality of the situation. Acquaintances and others in more distant associations may not be aware of the problem—or at least the more personal details.

Accepting some symptoms may be easier than accepting others. When visible symptoms such as sleeping and cataplexy occur in public, family and friends who are identified with the person may be embarrassed. Instead of reassuring the affected person, providing safety and comfort, and helping to smooth over the situation, they may act ashamed of the behavior—or ashamed of the person. This embarrassment may be interpreted as rejection, adding insult to injury.

Accepting the person's dropping off to sleep at any time at home is not always easy for the family either. They may continuously awaken the person and make sarcastic remarks in an effort to make the person feel guilty. What is needed is a little time and the family's approval to take a few short naps as needed. If others could realize that napping is part of the prescription for relieving sleepiness, it would help solve the problem.

The affected person's limited abilities to participate in family activities often creates dissension. Blame may be assessed and guilt incurred, especially when lack of participation is interpreted as lack of interest. If sleepiness prevents or interferes with driving times, it can wreak havoc on family schedules. Narcolepsy, especially EDS, takes a heavy toll on the family.

Only when others accept the person with all the abnormalities of the disorder can everyone start to work solving other problems.

Cooperation

The person with narcolepsy needs physical assistance as well as moral support. Anyone who must make lifestyle changes in order to cope with a disability faces insurmountable obstacles without the cooperation of those most closely involved.

One of the prevailing symptoms is chronic fatigue. This leaves the person continuously tired and without the energy or motivation to do many of the "old things" — including work and pleasure. Tired, sleepy people are often perceived as lazy — a trait likely to be met with antagonism and resentment. Instead of compassion and a helping hand, the person, who is so in need of relief, may be confronted with a stubborn refusal of assistance.

Without family cooperation, a person with narcolepsy has little hope of being able to cope with the disorder. The battle against the ravages of narcolepsy can either draw family members closer together or drive them apart. Sadly, many marriages end in broken homes.

Cooperation must also come from friends, co-workers, employers and teachers if a person with narcolepsy is to find success and satisfaction in this "new life." Since the doctor cannot educate everyone, the affected adult must learn to assume the role of educator and advocate. Before broaching the subject, some situations might benefit from a little advance planning. For example, before talking with an employer, consult with someone in business management as well as someone experienced in regard to narcolepsy (perhaps from a support group). As previously stated, parents must take that responsibility for their children.

Therapy Impairment

When positive support is poor or absent, the effectiveness of drug therapy is impaired. Symptoms typically become worse when the person is under stress and increasing the dosage is not going to solve the problem. Psychological trauma creates another whole set of problems to be dealt with.

Combined Effort

Able narcoleptics must form support groups and come to the aid of their own. Families must do their part. All these groups must join forces to form a support system to meet the needs of those suffering the effects of narcolepsy. Help must not only be available, it must be provided to the individual who may not be capable of reaching out for it. The question is, "Who will do the job?"

FOLLOW-UP TREATMENT

The following recommendations are made in the ASDA Consensus Statement:

1. A patient stabilized on stimulant medication should be seen by a physician at least once per year, and preferably once every six months, for assessment of the development of medication side effects including sleep disturbance, mood changes and cardiovascular or metabolic abnormalities.
2. Patients on pemoline should have liver function tests at the start of treatment, approximately four weeks after the initiation of treatment, at least once per year, and when there is any change in health that might suggest an alteration in liver function.
3. Polysomnographic reevaluation of patients with narcolepsy should be considered if there is a significant increase in symptoms of sleepiness or if there are specific symptoms suggesting new or increased sleep abnormalities as might occur in disorders such as sleep apnea or periodic limb movement disorder.
4. Continued prescription of stimulant medication by telephone or mail is not recommended if the patient has not been seen by the prescribing physician within the prior 18 months.

A COMPREHENSIVE PROGRAM
FOR THE MANAGEMENT OF SYMPTOMS

I. Good Doctor-Patient Relationship
II. Doctor Responsible for:
  A. Providing information on narcolepsy
  B. Prescribing/monitoring drug therapy
  C. Making referral to narcolepsy groups
  D. Counseling or making referral to counselor
    1. Teaching good communication skills
    2. Assisting with lifestyle adjustments
    3. Working with family members
    4. Advocating in employment issues, disability claims, etc.
III. Patient Responsible for (doctor provides info):
  A. Taking all medications *as directed*
  B. Taking therapeutic naps
  C. Developing healthful lifestyle
  D. Learning and using coping skills
IV. Combined effort of doctor-patient-family-others
  A. Psychosocial support:
     Understanding, Acceptance, Cooperation
  B. Practicing good communication skills

A good comprehensive management program needs to include all the above elements. Since most treatment nowadays includes only drug therapy, obviously it would be overwhelming for any doctor or sleep disorders center to implement a program of this magnitude immediately. However, it is a goal towards which they need to start working.

The rapidly expanding field of sleep disorders offers unlimited opportunities for those already in practice and for students now in medical school. The following Sociomedical Model of Counseling, developed by Dr. Meeta Goswami, offers an alternative to the traditional approach to patient management. This model is a narcoleptic's dream (but not of the hypnagogic variety). Instead of being a realistic fantasy, it could be a realistic solution to the problem of comprehensive management of symptoms.

SOCIOMEDICAL MODEL OF COUNSELING

Meeta Goswami, M.P.H., Ph.D., Director of The Narcolepsy Institute at Montefiore Medical Center in Bronx, New York, has developed a Sociomedical Model of Counseling. Developed specifically for narcolepsy, the concept may be applicable to other chronic illnesses as well. She outlines her model in "Psychosocial Aspects of Narcolepsy," edited by Goswami, et al.

Traditionally, the physician is the principal source of care, medical information and advice. The patient is a passive receiver of services. Such services include little attention in regard to how the medical condition impacts his/her life or what other support services may be needed.

Unlike the family doctor of the past, physicians now tend to specialize and restrict their observations to their areas of expertise. Consequently, a patient may be forced to consult a different doctor for each medical problem. Often there is no communication between the various care providers or between providers and patient. This depersonalized approach results in poor quality of care, and often discourages the patient to the point of discontinuing treatment.

Dr. Goswami's model recognizes that a combination of factors may contribute to, or result in, a medical condition. The doctor-patient relationship involves two-way communication, emphasizing patient feedback and involving the patient in the decision-making process.

A team approach is recommended. A physician would be responsible for the medical aspects, and a sociomedical counselor would be responsible for providing basic information on narcolepsy and total patient management of social, psychological, nutritional, and genetic concerns. By coordinating their activities, comprehensive medical and psychological aspects of care would be integrated and continuity of care would be maintained.

Patients with severe psychological or social problems requiring more intensive care would be referred to a specialist such as a psychologist, psychiatrist or social worker.

Dr. Goswami also advocates (1) minimal doses of stimulants and other medications to control any auxiliary symptoms, (2) therapeutic naps (short 10-20 minute naps) once or twice a day, (3) psychosocial support (acceptance, approval and cooperation from family, friends and business associates), and (4) referral to a local narcolepsy support group as well as to a national organization such as Narcolepsy Network, Inc.

MY EXPERIENCES WITH
DIAGNOSIS AND TREATMENT

IN 1961 (about three years after EDS had become a problem), I had a complete physical, primarily for the purpose of finding a cause and cure for my sleepiness. An EEG (electroencephalogram) showed I was having abnormal electrical storms in my brain, but at that time doctors did not associate them with narcolepsy. After a glucose tolerance test indicated I had low blood sugar, the doctor made a diagnosis of hypoglycemia. A special diet was helpful, but my sleepy symptoms still persisted.

In 1963, a psychiatrist at the University of Illinois Health Service, where I was working, became the first of a long line of doctors to attempt treating my EDS. Actually, he was probably treating me for emotional problems or depression. (Sleep medicine was then in its infancy, and there was never a mention made of a sleep disorder called narcolepsy.)

The doctor wrote me a prescription for nicotinic acid. I have no idea why he chose that particular drug, but it proved to be a poor choice. Within twenty minutes of taking the first dose, my heart was pounding, I could scarcely breathe, and I was turning a beet red color from my shoulders up. A nurse in the clinic promptly gave me a shot of adrenalin, and I was soon back to normal with only a memory of a bad drug reaction. The doctor scratched that drug off the list of possibilities and wrote me a prescription for Dexedrine. I remained on that stimulant for the next three years.

Soon afterwards, I moved to Austin and enrolled at The University of Texas. When I went to the Health Center to get a prescription for Dexedrine, I was quickly signed on as a patient in their Mental Health Department. I was scheduled to see one of their psychiatric interns every two weeks for psychotherapy to try to determine what deep, dark secret I was trying to escape through the defense mechanism of sleep.

Their interns worked on a rotation schedule, so every three months I had to start over with a new therapist. When I started on the third one (or he started on me), I quit—through or not.

On one of my first visits, the doctor decided to find out how I would respond to a tranquilizer rather than a stimulant. It was a knock-out on round one, and we crossed tranquilizers off the list.

Three years later (three months before graduation), an aunt sent me a magazine article about narcolepsy. It described every one of my symptoms—even ones I did not know were related. I immediately made an appointment with a doctor mentioned in the article. He listened to an accounting of my symptoms and, then and there, announced that I had a classic case of narcolepsy. Before I left his office, he wrote me a prescription for Ritalin instead of Dexedrine.

The following summer I remember as "The Summer of the Cataplectic Attack." It struck with a vengeance! After taking Ritalin for a year, it was beginning to lose some of its effectiveness. When this happens, doctors usually increase the dosage or suggest that you take a drug holiday (time off drugs—not good time on drugs). I opted for the holiday, but it was no picnic!

Back in those days, Ritalin was used to control both EDS and cataplexy. When I discontinued the Ritalin, the frequency and intensity of both symptoms increased. Now I realize I was suffering rebound cataplexy brought on by the sudden and complete withdrawal from the drug. (The only other time my attacks were that severe was when I stopped taking Desoxyn in 1971.) The continuing severe cataplectic attacks left me drained and depressed.

After several weeks of intense cataplexy, I called my doctor. He increased my dosage of Ritalin from 20 mg three times a day to 40 mg three times a day and told me to stay on it regularly. I followed doctor's orders and my symptoms were immediately back under control.

Ritalin was never a good drug for me. However, it was better than the Dexedrine. It was only moderately effective in keeping me awake and even then it produced an abnormal feeling of alertness. I think it was in some way responsible for my occultic dreaming, it caused me to have double vision (especially when watching TV), and it definitely caused a furry-type growth on my tongue.

Ritalin has the side effect of being an appetite suppressant and it did help me lose weight. If that had been the only benefit, it would not have been worth it. I virtually couldn't eat anything all day until the effects wore off in the evening.

I spent the summer of 1970 preparing for my fellowship year which was to begin in the fall. My biggest priority was to get on a more effective drug treatment program that would allow me to drive across the United States.

I called my doctor and he sent me a prescription for Desoxyn, better known to the public by the street name *speed.* He included detailed written instructions on how to take the drug. After trying it for two weeks, I called the doctor again and told him my head felt like it was going to split open. His response was to refer me to another doctor.

When I called the other doctor and explained the situation to him, he immediately exclaimed, "He has you on the wrong form of the drug!" This doctor assured me he could have me "living a normal life" within one week.

I saw this doctor in his office twice a day for four weeks. He changed my prescription to the other form of Desoxyn and increased my dosage to 120 mg a day. When I couldn't sleep at night, he prescribed 30 mg of Dalmane and forbade me to take any naps during the day. When I started hyperventilating, he placed me on 20 mg of Valium.

At the end of the month, I was out of both time and money. But I was far from being "normalized." Quite to the contrary, my mental state had deteriorated to the point that I was almost dysfunctional. Nevertheless, as I had to get on with my life, the doctor dismissed me with instructions to regulate the dosages myself and recommended that I see a psychiatrist. He also wrote me a letter saying he didn't appreciate my complications (whatever that meant).

Four months later, I gave up my fellowship. And, while still under the influence of prescription drugs, I remarried. Immediately, my husband encouraged me to go off all drugs. He didn't want me to take a drug holiday—he wanted me off drugs permanently. He thought I needed to get them out of my system and give my body a rest. I agreed very reluctantly, more because of the severe cataplectic attacks than the excessive sleepiness. The first step was to cut down my dosage of Desoxyn. Then I stopped the Dalmane and threw the Valium in the trash. A few months later, I flushed the last seven hundred 5 mg tablets of Desoxyn down the toilet! (At street prices, that would have amounted to a nice chunk of change.)

I certainly am not suggesting that anyone else follow my example of going off all medications. Any withdrawal should be done gradually and under the care of a doctor. Besides that, what is right for one is not necessarily right for another. Circumstances must also be considered. It was my change in marital status that made it possible for me to go off drugs, since I no longer had to support myself.

For fourteen years I stayed off drugs and at home. I was so busy taking care of children and an invalid mother that I had little time for anything else. After Mother died and the children were gone, I read about Cylert in *The Eye Opener*, the newsletter of the late American Narcolepsy Association. The time was right in my life and I decided to give it a try.

My first prescription was for 18.75 mg, which i⸍ ⸍he minimum daily dosage. During the eight years I hav⸍ on the drug, I have increased the dosage twice—first ⸍ and then to the present level of 56.25 mg. I take dosage about 8:30 every morning and don't take any more during the day. Any increase in amount or taking it later in the day increases my difficulty in sleeping at night.

Cylert is a mild stimulant, and the most natural-acting one I have taken. I have experienced very few bad side effects, and most of them occur only when I take a larger-than-regular dosage (perhaps to keep me awake for some special occasion). Then I may have heart palpitations or I may become very agitated or temperamental. When I feel this effect coming on, I give my husband fair warning.

After having taken Dexedrine, Ritalin and Desoxyn, I am content to be on Cylert. It is only moderately effective, but it enables me to do the things I need to do without having to endure the bad side effects the other drugs had for me. The biggest difference it makes in my life (as compared to no stimulant) is that it enables me to drive in town—and in Dallas that covers a lot of territory. I still can't stay awake in church and passive situations. But there is much I *can* do—like write a book!

CAUTION: I have given you my own feelings about my own experiences with certain drugs. Keep in mind that responses to different drugs and dosages of drugs varies with each individual. There is no way to predict what drug will be most effective for a certain person. Trial and error is the only way to know.

I included this information because my experiences illustrate many of the problems involved in managing drug therapy. Virtually everyone has problems of one kind or another. The process is—let's face it—a hassle. But it is worth the effort if it helps to bring our symptoms under satisfactory control and enables us to live a satisfying life.

12
NARCOLEPSY IN CHILDREN

SINCE NARCOLEPSY is a genetic disorder, parents *should* be the ones to detect any symptoms that develop in their children. Unfortunately, many parents who have narcolepsy are still searching for a correct diagnosis of their own symptoms.

The first problem is lack of knowledge about all disorders of excessive daytime sleepiness and difficulty in getting a correct diagnosis. The second is that families are largely unaware that disorders of EDS are inheritable. Thirdly, even if someone has been diagnosed with narcolepsy or some other EDS disorder, they frequently fail to contact other family members (grown children, siblings, aunts, uncles and cousins) to inform them of the potential for others having or developing some form of EDS. Consequently, families don't know to be "on the lookout" for signs in their children.

When narcolepsy does occur in children, teachers are often the first to observe the symptom of excessive daytime sleepiness. Unfortunately, teachers are often antagonized by students sleeping in class. If they are not knowledgeable about narcolepsy, teachers may attribute sleeping in class to a variety of other reasons, such as not enough sleep at night, laziness, stupidity, disinterest in school work, etc. Children's efforts to overcome sleepiness may be misunderstood and labeled as behavior problems.

If the problem is not identified and the child does not receive help, grades will begin to drop. Subsequently, a pattern of failure and lowered self-esteem begins to develop.

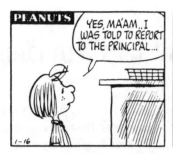

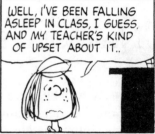

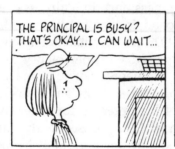

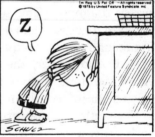

"Unfortunately, teachers are often antagonized by students sleeping in class."

Perhaps this is the saddest of all the consequences of narcolepsy. If parents are notified their child is sleeping in class, they should make an immediate effort to determine the cause. If a diagnosis of narcolepsy is made, they need to report this information to the school and schedule appointments (jointly if possible) with all teachers, the school counselor and the school nurse. It is the parents' responsibility to make sure school personnel understand their child's symptom(s) and how they can affect behavior and grades. However, if the parents *cannot* or *will not* assume that responsibility, a teacher or counselor must follow through with appropriate action.

Ask for teacher-staff cooperation in assuring your child gets any additional help and/or special considerations that may be necessary. This pertains to extra-curricular activities as well as coursework. All concerned adults need to monitor the child's interactions with others to be sure social adjustment is progressing satisfactorily. If it becomes apparent this cooperation is lacking or school authorities have some doubt regarding your child's disabilities due to narcolepsy, the attending physician may need to intercede on behalf of the student. The counselor especially needs to be aware of the psychosocial aspects of narcolepsy. It is imperative neither the child's grades nor his/her self-esteem suffer due to the consequences of narcolepsy.

Children are bombarded with other problems in addition to their learning difficulties. They are embarrassed by being different from their peers and likely will make vain attempts to hide their condition. Or they may make up stories in an effort to explain their sometimes odd behaviors. They are likely frightened by their symptoms and unable to understand and accept them. They may be especially terrified if they experience hypnagogic hallucinations, sleep paralysis and/or cataplexy. These are experiences which even their parents cannot understand (unless, of course, one of them has narcolepsy).

A support group, or even one other individual who has narcolepsy, can be extremely helpful in reassuring the child. A professional counselor, *who understands narcolepsy*, can help the child to make the many difficult adjustments demanded by the disorder.

Career counseling is crucial for children and young people with narcolepsy. The basis for future plans must be laid early through an understanding and acceptance of the fact that there are certain limitations imposed by the disorder. Occupations in which EDS and/or cataplexy might prove to be potentially hazardous to themselves and/or others should be ruled out. Such job-types might include airline pilot, air controller, surgeon, truck driver, heavy equipment operator and high rise construction worker. Active-duty police workers and firefighters are other risky occupations. (Summer jobs are also affected.)

Hopefully, symptoms could be controlled sufficiently to allow the performance of any type of work. Realistically, such might not be the case. Or a person may have only mild excessive daytime sleepiness when deciding on a career only to find that the symptom worsens or that cataplexy develops at a later date.

It is far better for young people to face reality and work toward a suitable profession than it is for them to meet with failure or rejection after years of preparation in the wrong field. If good viable employment alternatives are offered and young people receive the support and encouragement they need, it should not be a big problem.

One of the biggest priorities for all those concerned with narcolepsy at any level should be ways of identifying narcolepsy when it exists in young children. The sooner it can be diagnosed and treated, the better adjusted and more normal their lives will be. Children are probably the most victimized by the disorder. Many are doomed to a lifetime of failure unless they get the help they need. Otherwise, they must struggle desperately against the odds to succeed.

13
UNDERSTANDING NARCOLEPSY

A N UNDERSTANDING of the nature of narcolepsy is dependent upon a basic understanding of normal sleep and its processes. Actually, we know very little about this mysterious realm of sleep in which we spend about one third of our lives. In the past, sleep was thought to be a passive state in which the body rested. Now it is known that rest and restoration are accomplished during sleep, but the body and brain must work very hard to do the job.

Since the early 1960's, when sleep medicine had its beginnings, researchers have made great strides in identifying some of the processes occurring during sleep. Knowledge about the kinds of sleep and the stages of sleep and sleep cycles is of particular interest to an understanding of narcolepsy.

There are two kinds of sleep and five distinct stages of sleep identified by electroencephalogram (EEG) brain wave recordings. The two kinds of sleep are: REM (rapid eye movement) sleep and NREM (non-rapid eye movement) sleep. REM refers both to the kind of sleep and to the stage of sleep in which it occurs. NREM refers only to the kind of sleep; it occurs in all the other four stages of sleep.

NORMAL SLEEP

A normal eight-hour sleep period is divided into four or five cycles (depending upon how long a person sleeps), each lasting approximately ninety minutes. Within these cycles, the stages of sleep occur in sequential order, but not all stages are present in each cycle. The stages which do occur vary in duration from cycle-to-cycle within the course of the sleep period. The first cycle contains all five stages in orderly sequence, but subsequent cycles contain progressively less sleep in Stages 2, 3 and 4 and correspondingly more sleep is devoted to Stage 1 and REM.

A drowsy wakefulness with accompanying *Alpha waves* begins the prelude to sleep. From there we start a descent into sleep which progresses rapidly through the light sleep of Stage 1 and into Stage 2, where true sleep begins. About half of adult sleep is spent in this stage. We quickly drift down into Stage 3 and then Stage 4, which are the periods of deepest sleep. A large portion of our sleep during the first half of the night is spent in Stage 4 sleep, especially if we are tired or sleep deprived. From Stage 4 we begin drifting up into Stage 3 and then Stage 2.

RAPID EYE MOVEMENT (REM) SLEEP

When we emerge from Stage 2, we are not back where we started, but in a special stage referred to as REM sleep. This stage begins about ninety minutes after sleep onset. (For people with narcolepsy it can begin almost immediately.)

In REM sleep, brain wave patterns become similar to those in the waking state. The mind is very alert — not to the outside world — but to the activities being experienced in the world of dreams. Eyes dart about behind closed lids as though following a drama as it unfolds; thus the term *rapid eye movement*. REM sleep is known as the dreaming stage, but some dreaming also occurs during NREM.

REM periods grow progressively longer in each one of the four or five sleep cycles. In the first cycle, REM sleep lasts about ten minutes; in the second cycle about twenty minutes. In the third, fourth and fifth cycles, REM sleep may last as long as forty or sixty minutes.

REM sleep is believed to have an important function in consolidating memory as part of the learning process. People deprived of REM tend to learn less effectively and become irritable and anxious. Narcoleptics apparently get as much REM sleep as the normal population, but the problem is with mistiming of REM episodes.

NARCOLEPTIC SLEEP: REM—KEY TO UNDERSTANDING

Remember, REM sleep is the key to understanding narcolepsy. Although the different symptoms may seem to be unrelated, most of them are fragments of REM sleep cropping up at the wrong time. Remember, too, that REM sleep, occurring normally about ninety minutes into the sleep cycle, is accompanied by sleep paralysis. Narcoleptics are sometimes aware of this phenomenon when REM sleep occurs immediately upon sleep onset or upon awakening, when the brain is only partially asleep. Similar paralysis is experienced as loss of muscle control during cataplectic attacks. Precise connections between these different occurrences is not yet known.

14
CAUSES OF NARCOLEPSY

RESEARCH ON NARCOLEPSY, conducted primarily in university and hospital-related facilities, continues to search for the causes and ultimately a cure for the disorder. The major areas of focus are:

FAMILIAL TRAIT (Inherited)

Narcolepsy is a genetic disorder. The predisposition for narcolepsy can be inherited. Anyone diagnosed with narcolepsy should make information available to relatives and attempt to determine if other members are affected. Medical genealogy can be an important factor in identifying families affected by disorders of excessive daytime sleepiness. EDS appears more frequently in families than does narcolepsy. For a first degree relative of a narcoleptic, the risk of developing some disorder of excessive sleepiness is eight times greater than for the general population. The method by which the predisposition to inheriting narcolepsy is transmitted is unknown, but research is shedding some light on the subject.

GENETIC COMPONENT

It appears there might be several genes that predispose a person to narcolepsy. A person with one or more of these genes might develop narcolepsy, whereas a person without any of the narcolepsy genes will not develop it.

ENVIRONMENTAL FACTORS

Whether or not someone with a genetic predisposition to narcolepsy will develop it depends upon a wide range of environmental factors. Particular factors, which may be different for each individual, have not been identified. In general, viruses, bacteria, chemicals and even psychological stress are suspect.

GENETIC MARKERS FOR NARCOLEPSY

Almost everyone who has narcolepsy has a specific blood type known as HLA-DR2. HLA stands for Human Leucocyte Antigen, a family of proteins critical to the immune system. The DR2 gene is a key component of the HLA system that controls the body's immune defenses. Most people with DR2 have the closely related gene DQB1-0602, which is actually a better marker for narcolepsy.

Although an estimated 20–30% of the general population carries DR2 and/or DQB1-0602, only a tiny fraction will ever develop narcolepsy. Researchers theorize that other unidentified genes and probably environmental factors are needed in addition to the HLA factors to cause the onset of narcolepsy. The high correlation between the DR2 and the DQB1-0602 genes and narcolepsy suggests they code for a predisposition to the disorder. This association also suggests narcolepsy may be an autoimmune disorder (see page 85).

NEUROTRANSMITTERS

Millions of neurons (brain cells) communicate with each other by means of chemicals called neurotransmitters. If any part of this complex system of sending and receiving messages is not functioning properly, the desired action will not take place.

Research studies suggest the brain may be hypersensitive to the neurotransmitter acetylcholine, which is important in the control of REM sleep. Other biochemical studies involve neurotransmitters called monoamines (dopamine, norepinephrine and serotonin), which are important for the regulation of sleep, arousal and alertness. Stimulants and antidepressants are thought to work by enhancing the effects of these neurotransmitters. Research on monoamines and how current narcolepsy drugs act on them may lead to the development of better treatments. Ultimately, however, the discovery of the genes that initially produce the acetylcholine and monoamine imbalances could result in finding a total cure for narcolepsy rather than treatment that only reduces the symptoms of the disorder.

AUTOIMMUNE HYPOTHESIS

Although there is no direct evidence to support the hypothesis, factors (such as the HLA-DR2 marker) suggest narcolepsy might be an autoimmune disorder. The body's immune system provides protection against foreign objects. Occasionally, for some reason it attacks its own tissue, usually causing significant damage. Hypothetically, in narcolepsy, the area in the brain that controls the sleep/wake processes could be damaged as a result of this kind of immune attack.

15
A Personal Note on Coping

NARCOLEPSY IS incurable. However, it is not hopeless. Drug treatment is helpful to a degree, but overall it can be rated as only moderately effective. Therefore, we narcoleptics must learn to live as best we can with this monster that threatens to gobble up our most productive waking hours. In large part, our success or failure depends on us.

Coping skills for us equate to survival tactics under wartime conditions! Considering this fact, we must prepare ourselves with the best weapons at our disposal—starting with knowledge. Those of us who are affected (both directly and indirectly) need to know and understand the basic facts about the disorder, as well as available treatment, research and legislation concerning our welfare.

How does such information help us to cope better with narcolepsy? Speaking for myself, I think it helps me to see the overall picture instead of my one little piece. I know that I am not in this alone—there are about 149,999 other Americans in the same boat!

Knowing the facts helps to reassure me that I am an intelligent person. Although I may have a few mental handicaps, I am not dumb. Neither am I a dummy because I walk around like a zombie some of the time. It helps me to know that I am not inherently lazy because I have little energy and often need to sleep. And anything that builds a little self-confidence and self-esteem goes a long way.

Knowlege about the medications being used to treat narcolepsy means that I can be a participating member, along with my doctor, in my management program. Armed with current information and a good dose of self-esteem, I can communicate my needs, reactions and feelings to my doctor.

Knowledge about legislation means I can act as an informed citizen to help protect my rights in regard to job, disability, insurance, driver's license, and the procurement of the drugs I need.

Knowledge, along with the self-confidence it generates, helps me to tell others about narcolepsy and how it impacts my life. I might mention here some good advice my mother gave me: "Don't ever tell a lie—but you don't always have to tell everything you know." The dangers of openly acknowledging your narcolepsy are very real and much may be at risk. So be discerning in who you tell, how much you tell, when you tell, and why. All information might not be appropriate or necessary in all situations.

Personally, I see a great deal of merit in telling others I have narcolepsy. One reason I mention narcolepsy is in the interest of public education. Many people have never heard of narcolepsy; those who have heard of it may not know what it is. Another probable reason for openness is to offer an excuse for falling asleep (if I do) or for any other strange symptom(s) that I may exhibit, or for something I may not be able to do.

In addition to knowledge about narcolepsy, there are many other things that we can do to help ourselves deal with the obstacles presented by the disorder. Just as there is no 100% effective drug to control symptoms, neither is there a coping tool for every problem. Nevertheless, by using our resources to the best of our abilities, we can improve our circumstances. It is not the changes of lifestyle forced upon us nor the sacrifices demanded of us that affect our quality of life as much as our attitudes. With knowledge, a good positive attitude and determination, we can surmount the obstacles.

Self-Help Guide

Attitudes

- Accept yourself as a person with narcolepsy. You are different in some ways and you have some special needs. That's OK.
- Don't be ashamed of your condition or its symptoms. You have no more need to apologize for your actions than a heart or cancer patient would for theirs. Sure, there may be embarrassing situations, but don't agonize over them.
- Develop a good sense of humor. It's much nicer to have people laughing with you than at you, and it can sometimes help you to "save face." In any case, it makes life much more pleasant.
- Don't be too hard on yourself. Set realistic goals that you can accomplish. Don't push yourself beyond your limits and then be your own worst critic. If you are a perfectionist, rethink your priorities. Is it better to complete every task perfectly or to be well-adjusted and content—and let others be also?
- Don't be too easy on yourself either. Don't allow yourself to use narcolepsy as a crutch—an excuse for not doing the things you can and should do.
- Don't feel guilty because of things beyond your control. Do the best you can with what you have and accept that from yourself.
- Accentuate the positive and eliminate the negative. Think on the good side, and be thankful for what you have rather than complaining about what could have been.

OUTSIDE HELP

☐ See a sleep disorders specialist. Assure yourself insofar as possible that you have received a correct diagnosis. Work with your doctor to achieve an effective drug therapy program.

☐ Get a good physical examination to determine if there are any physical problems contributing to your condition. If there are, do what you can to correct them.

☐ Discuss with your doctor whether or not you need additional counseling for emotional problems. Many sleep disorder centers have staff psychiatrists or psychologists. Or they may refer you to a good counselor *who is familiar with the problems of narcolepsy.*

Inform yourself about the different types of counseling available and determine what best meets your needs. You may not need in-depth psychotherapy delving back into your childhood and the dark niches of your psyche. Brief therapy, which is usually limited to less than a dozen sessions, is gaining in acceptance and can be very effective. There is a need and a purpose for various approaches.

☐ Join a narcolepsy support group. If there isn't one in your area, consider starting one. Even having one other person with narcolepsy to talk to can be a tremendous help.

☐ Join Narcolepsy Network, Inc. Request that your name be put on the mailing list for *Sleep Health*, the newsletter published by the National Sleep Foundation (NSF). These organizations can keep you updated on news of interest concerning narcolepsy, work on your behalf to protect your rights and advocate for you.

☐ Develop a good rapport with your pharmacist. He can counsel you on new drugs, side effects, drug interactions, and assist you in obtaining the drugs you need. It is often in your best interests to use one pharmacy for all your prescriptions—even if it means paying a little bit more.

PRACTICAL PRACTICES

☐ Live a healthful lifestyle, which includes:
- Good nutritional habits. Watch for foods that worsen daytime sleep; those that keep you awake at night.
- *Regular* eating habits
  - ☐ Eat meals on a regular schedule.
  - ☐ Don't eat lunch too late — at the time of maximum sleepiness.
  - ☐ Don't skip meals and then snack on junk foods. This may be of particular concern if you are on a drug that acts as an appetite suppressant.
- Weight control
  - ☐ Enlist the help of someone to whom you can be accountable.
  - ☐ Switch to low calorie/nonfat or low-fat foods; fruit and veggie snacks.
  - ☐ Don't keep rich, tempting foods on hand. Ask your family's cooperation.
- Limited amounts of caffeine (coffee, tea and chocolate). Switch to decaffeinated drinks in the afternoon.
- No tobacco (cigarettes, plug or pipe). Smoking can be exceptionally dangerous to the health of those who fall asleep with a cigarette in their hand.
- Moderate amounts or no alcohol. Don't mix alcohol with certain drugs. Check with your pharmacist if in doubt.
- Adequate exercise. Walking at least three times a week is highly recommended; no strenuous exercise just before bedtime.
- Good, regular sleeping habits.
  - ☐ Go to bed and get up at the same time every day.
  - ☐ Get enough sleep to meet your needs.
  - ☐ Be comfortable. (Good bed; room temperature not too hot or cold, etc.)

□ Take short naps (10–20 minutes) 1–3 times a day as needed. Short naps help to maintain alertness; long naps are more apt to leave you feeling groggy. Some people find a longer nap after lunch beneficial.

□ Try not to sleep so much during the day that it will interfere with your nighttime sleep.

□ Do important or tedious tasks during alert periods; stimulating tasks at sleepy times of day.

SPECIFIC HELPS

Taking Drugs

□ Take all medication as directed and on schedule.

□ Report all medications to your doctor.

WARNING: Before you receive any anesthetics (even Novocain or nitrous oxide at a dentist's office), be sure the doctor and the anesthetist know you have narcolepsy. Do not assume they know you are (or may be) very sensitive to anesthetics and may have difficulty coming out from under the influence of such drugs. Provide information on all drugs you are taking.

□ Watch for side effects and drug interactions that could worsen your condition or prove dangerous.

□ Read labels on over-the-counter drugs, such as antihistamines that cause drowsiness; pain or cold medications that act as stimulants. Ask the pharmacist to help find medicines best suited to your condition.

Safety

□ Practice the "Code of Caution." Just as faithfully as we obey the rules of the road, we need to observe the danger signs for narcolepsy. Many activities both on and off the job should have flashing yellow caution lights for narcoleptics. Some should even have red lights. Others require patience while waiting for the green light. This is especially true for those affected by cataplexy. We dare not ignore certain risks to ourselves and/or others. We must exercise good judgment.

☐ Use the Buddy System. It can be your best friend. There are many activities that we can continue to enjoy as long as we have someone with us. Hopefully, that person could handle any emergency but, if not, at least you would have someone who could call for help.

Never swim alone. (Some people report plunging into cold water brings on a cataplectic attack.) Perform a mental safety check before undertaking any activity by yourself. Don't take chances if it could prove dangerous to yourself or others.

☐ Don't act as "the buddy" for someone else in potentially dangerous situations. Don't assume the position of responsible party when you may not be able to do the job. For example, don't take children swimming by yourself. Even if there is a lifeguard or someone else nearby, you might not be alert enough or capable of summoning help.

☐ Carry a narcolepsy identification card in your billfold. (Optional: if you have cataplexy, you can include a description on the back.)

Cataplectic Attack

☐ Prepare the people who are most likely to be with you, in advance. Help them to understand what is happening during an attack and what to expect. Let them know you are conscious during these times, how you feel, and how they can help you—be specific. Do you want to be touched or left alone? Will you be likely to need support?

If you have a total body collapse, should they help you sit down or lie down—on the floor if necessary? How long might the attack last? Might you sleep or cry afterwards?

These questions need to be thought out, discussed and answered in advance. You can save yourself and

---

NARCOLEPSY PATIENT:

_____

Narcolepsy is a neurological sleep disorder. The main
symptom is excessive sleepiness. My other symptoms
include: _____

_____

See back for description of cataplexy.*
My doctor is: _____
Phone: _____
I am taking the following drugs for this condition:

_____

- -

* Cataplexy is a sudden, brief paralysis of voluntary
muscles, usually triggered by strong emotion. It is in no
way related to epilepsy. During a cataplectic attack the
person remains conscious and aware of what is going on.
Attacks usually pass within a few minutes; if prolonged,
the person may go to sleep and start dreaming. Speech
may be garbled or impossible. Provide any necessary
support or help in sitting or lying down. Be sure the head
is in a position to allow proper breathing. Give reassurance
and wait for the attack to pass.

Sample narcolepsy identification card

others a great deal of anxiety and embarrassment by
being prepared.

□ Keep outwardly calm. If you panic, you can imagine what
others will do.

□ Focus on remaining inwardly calm. Forget whatever
emotion brought on the attack—don't think about it.
Think *calm*—act *calm*—be *calm*—and stay *calm* until the
attack subsides.

☐ Sometimes (if possible and if there is enough time) the best thing to do might be to get away from whatever it is that is triggering the attack.

☐ When it's over—it's over! If your head fell in your plate, wipe the egg off your face and go on about your business.

Hypnagogic Hallucinations

☐ Leave a small night light on so the room is not in total darkness.

☐ Reassure yourself that all doors are locked and the house is secure before you go to bed.

☐ Close all closet doors. (Very important to some)

☐ Don't watch horror stories on TV or at the movies; don't read horror stories. They may come back to haunt you in your dreams.

Driving

☐ Coordinate taking your stimulant with your driving times. Take it long enough in advance that it will be effective when you start out. Plan to stop before it wears off.

☐ If you cannot always count on being alert at the appointed time(s), avoid regularly scheduled driving by yourself. If you have an appointment or someone is depending on you at a certain time, you may be tempted to drive when you shouldn't.

☐ Take a short nap before starting out.

☐ Have a driving partner who can relieve you.

☐ If you have to wait (such as in the doctor's office) take a nap so you will be ready to drive home.

☐ If you get sleepy while driving:

■ Stop and take a short nap. Stop in a safe place, lock your car doors, roll up the windows except for a little ventilation. Keep a timer or travel alarm in the car so you won't oversleep.

- Stop and walk around; get something to drink and/or eat.
- If you absolutely can't stop, turn on the air conditioner and/or roll down your window.
- Turn the music up loud and sing along.
- Memorize poetry or scripture; clip reference material to your sun visor. Be loud, dramatic and eloquent—really ham it up!
- Carry cold drinks and ice in a cooler. Put some ice in a cloth to bathe your face and/or the back of your neck.

Working

☐ IF you are in what could be considered a hazardous occupation AND you cannot get good control over your symptoms of EDS and cataplexy, you seriously need to consider changing jobs. Don't take chances with your life and that of others.

☐ Tell someone you work with that you have narcolepsy and describe your symptoms. Use discretion as to whom you tell and how much you reveal, but it is important that someone close to you know about your condition.

☐ Do important and/or tedious, boring tasks while you are most alert; save more stimulating ones for sleepy times. (This advice is worth repeating.)

☐ If you feel drowsy, take a short break. Go to the restroom, splash cold water on your face, get something to drink, do exercises (walk up and down a few flights of stairs); take a nap!

☐ Change activities—make phone calls, run errands. Don't abuse or misuse time in the process.

Organizational Skills

Being organized is another way of compensating for several problems experienced by narcoleptics, namely:

☐ A sleepy, confused mind; inability to concentrate.

☐ Wasting time; making mistakes due to sleepiness.

☐ Memory impairment; forgetfulness.

☐ Procrastination.

☐ Difficulty in sticking with jobs to completion.

Planning and organizational skills can help you be more efficient and more accurate; thereby, saving time, stress — and maybe your job! Becoming a more efficient person should also make you feel better about yourself — and that's important.

Here are a few suggestions:

☐ Keep a planning calendar. Fill in birthdays and other annual events first. Then take one month at a time, filling in dates as they come to your attention.

☐ Prepare a daily list of "Things to Do Today." Set your priorities so that the most important things will get done first. Be realistic and not idealistic. Delegate jobs to others when appropriate instead of trying to do everything yourself.

☐ Have a separate "Projects List" of things that need to be done or that you want to do as time allows. Keep it posted in a convenient place (such as on a bulletin board or refrigerator) for quick reference.

☐ Keep a shopping list or lists — perhaps one for groceries; another for household items, etc. Don't forget your list(s) when you go shopping.

☐ Schedule routine tasks such as grocery shopping, cleaning house, washing and ironing (and whatever things men do) at regular times.

☐ Have "a place for everything and everything in its place." Make it a habit to put things where they belong every time, and you will spend less time hunting for them later.

☐ Keep note pads handy at all times and use them. Transfer important info to calendars, files, etc.

☐ Schedule passive, sleep-inducing tasks during your most alert times and active tasks during "sleepy" times of day.

- [ ] Use a timer (with a loud ringer) to wake you from short naps and to remind you of things to do during the day.

Teacher-Student Communication (for Adults)

Before the first class, inform the teacher that you have a sleep disorder. Take a brochure about narcolepsy and point out that sleepiness can be uncontrollable. Ask that you not be embarrassed if you get sleepy or fall asleep in class. Ask permission to stand at the back of the room at times to help maintain alertness.

Study Skills

- [ ] Schedule reading/studies for your most alert time of day.
- [ ] Take a short nap before starting to read/study.
- [ ] Keep a timer handy. You may need to take several mininaps over a long study period.
- [ ] *Stop* when concentration becomes an effort and/or your eyes have trouble focusing on the material. You *must* do something to bring yourself back to a state of alertness. Continuing on in that condition is generally a waste of time. It may even do more harm than good if you continue your efforts while in automatic behavior.
- [ ] Take a short break or change activities to help break the "spell." Stretch, exercise, walk.... If nothing else works, take a short nap.
- [ ] Keep the room relatively cool; perhaps use a fan to keep the air circulating.
- [ ] Sit in a straight chair at a desk or table. Don't get too comfortably settled in an easy chair.
- [ ] Choose a place that is brightly lit. Use the brightest light bulbs suitable for lamp or fixtures.
- [ ] Don't put off studying until the last minute. You may not be able to stay awake and the pressure will only make it worse.

16
SUPPORT GROUPS

A SUPPORT GROUP can be crucial in helping people cope with the symptoms and the consequences of narcolepsy. We all need to be understood and accepted as we are. People with narcolepsy are no exception.

What do you do after the doctor diagnoses your condition, prescribes a drug or drugs to help control your symptoms — and then sends you home? How do you learn to live with this incurable, life-long condition that changes your life forever? The majority of people with narcolepsy probably "go it alone" except, perhaps, for the help of a spouse or close friend. But there is no help quite like that which comes from someone else who "has been there."

It is not uncommon for a person to have the disorder for ten or twenty years and never have had the opportunity to talk to another narcoleptic. If and when that first conversation comes, it is like opening up the flood gates. Relief is probably the biggest emotion. What a relief to know there is someone else in the world who really understands what you go through and how you feel! Even if you never have another such experience, at least you know you are not alone in your struggle with this disorder.

The primary purpose of narcolepsy support groups is to provide an opportunity for people with similar problems to get together and share experiences, discuss their problems and hopefully find some solutions, express their feelings, and obtain information. Family members and friends (who often serve as drivers) are welcome. Spouses usually attend meetings, since they are often in as much need of help as the one with narcolepsy. Meetings sometimes have separate groups for family members, who have their own set of problems to discuss.

In addition, support groups can act as a contact and referral source, engage in public education projects, and become politically active in supporting legislation and protecting the rights of people with narcolepsy.

Generally, there are three types of groups:

□ Those sponsored by a medical group such as a sleep disorders center.
□ Those run by people with narcolepsy.
□ Those run by a combination of the above.

It is perhaps easier to start a group under the auspices of a medical group. Usually they will provide mailings to their patients, provide the meeting place and provide the refreshments. However, there are other considerations, namely, that other doctors do not want to send their patients to a meeting at another medical facility. For that reason, it is often preferable for the group to dissociate itself from any particular group of professionals. Another consideration is the fact that patients benefit more from a group in which they are active participants.

In areas where there are several sleep disorders facilities, a group might want to schedule a meeting at each place and ask a representative of that facility to speak. There is a two-fold advantage to members of the medical profession visiting or participating in a support group. Not only do members benefit from the wisdom of the professionals, but the professionals have an opportunity to observe and learn from those who live in the real world of narcolepsy. Since doctors cannot release the names and addresses of their patients, they are usually cooperative in mailing notices of group meetings.

Narcolepsy support groups usually meet no more than once a month or quarterly. Some groups meet only once or twice a year. They may meet in a public facility such as a library, school or church; or they may meet in a private home. If meeting in a private home, use discernment and caution in publicly announcing the location.

If you are planning to start a new group, you should be aware of some built-in problems. Narcoleptics are not the best people in the world to attend meetings on a regular basis. Part of their problem is not having the motivation to want to do things. Of course, the other part to that is not having the energy to do even the things they want to do. Some have memory problems and may forget the meeting. Others cannot drive and are dependent upon friends and relatives for transportation. Taking all this into consideration, most groups find it more satisfactory to meet less frequently.

Don't let all of that discourage you. The need for a group is vital! If you don't succeed at first, try, try again. Don't give up—it is well worth the effort. Try a publicity campaign to get the word out.

Here are some suggestions:

- Submit articles to the newspaper(s).
- Get meeting dates on community calendars.
- Contact all sleep disorders centers, doctors known to treat narcolepsy and your county medical association. Send them information about your group and ask them to refer inquiries to you or some other designated person.
- Participate in a local health fair. Pass out brochures on narcolepsy and information on your support group.
- Contact local radio and television stations. Request them to present information about narcolepsy. Call in to talk about narcolepsy on radio talk shows.

If you call in to a talk show, you can read a prepared statement if you are not comfortable speaking extemporaneously. If you say you are going to read something, you don't have to worry about *sounding like* you are reading, and you can be brief without forgetting anything. Keep the book open to "Basic Facts About Narcolepsy" in order to answer questions if you have the opportunity.

For information on sources to help in forming groups or in locating a group near you, see "Sources" on pages 157–158.

17
POLITICAL STATUS

SLEEPINESS AS A major national health problem was recognized by Congress in 1988 when it created the National Commission for Sleep Disorders Research. Acting on findings submitted by this commission, Congress established the National Center for Sleep Disorders Research (NCSDR) in 1993. The Center was placed within the National Heart, Lung and Blood Institute, which is part of the National Institutes of Health (NIH).

Its priorities will be: (1) to increase awareness about sleep disorders among health professionals and the general public, and (2) to foster basic and clinical research. Previously, sleep research funded by NIH was distributed throughout approximately five institutes. This new coordination of research projects will facilitate efforts and conserve funds.

However, even before the NCSDR was established, there was some difference of opinion as to what direction research should take. Should all funds be concentrated on finding a cure for narcolepsy? Or should some funds be allocated to improving or creating medications for interim treatment? (As a narcoleptic, it would be hard for me to remain silent on this issue. Hopefully a cure for narcolepsy will be found in the near future. Realistically, it may be a long way off. In the meantime, we need all the help we can get to live with this disorder — *NOW!*)

Diseases affecting less than 200,000 persons in this country are classified as *orphan diseases.* Although it is estimated that between 150,000 and 250,000 people have narcolepsy, less than 100,000 have been diagnosed. According to which statistics are used, narcolepsy could fall in or out of the group known as orphan diseases.

Narcolepsy Network, Inc. represents the disorder by membership in the National Organization for Rare Disorders (NORD). Since narcolepsy is a genetic disorder, it also shares common interests and concerns with the Alliance of Genetic Support Groups. Smaller groups which represent less common disorders have found it advantageous to band together for purposes of promoting legislation, research and organizational techniques.

Narcolepsy's best hope for recognition is to align itself with the other sleep disorders. Dr. William C. Dement, Chair of the National Commission on Sleep Disorders Research and Director of the Stanford University Sleep Disorders Center, states that there are over 40 million Americans who suffer from one or more chronic sleep disorders. In addition, millions more are sleep deprived. You would think that so many sleep-affected people would be able to command attention!

The problem, as reported by Dr. Dement, is getting the word into the medical schools and out to the public. Modern sleep disorders medicine is a relatively new field, but one of major importance to the well-being and quality of life of the American people.

My mother was a visiting teacher and worked with disadvantaged families for years. She frequently came across children with head lice and this is what she told them: "It isn't a disgrace to have lice, but it is a disgrace to keep them." (Then she helped them to eliminate the problem.) This thinking (and action) could be very appropriately applied to the problem of sleep disorders. When we didn't know the problem existed, it wasn't a national disgrace to have it. But now that we know the enormity of the situation—and have the potential to do something about it—it is a disgrace to allow it to continue.

18
BENEFITS
AND LEGAL MATTERS

DISABILITY BENEFITS

IF YOUR NARCOLEPSY is so severe that you are unable to get
or hold a job, you may be eligible for one or more of the
following disability benefits. For information on these programs, contact your local Social Security office.

Social Security Disability Insurance (SSDI) provides
monthly cash benefits for disabled workers and their de-
pendents. It covers those who have contributed to the Social
Security Trust Fund through payroll taxes, and the monthly
benefit is based on individual earnings. Unlike workman's
compensation, the worker does not have to be disabled on
the job in order to qualify. Children under 18 also qualify
for SSDI if their disability is severe enough that, as an adult,
they would not be able to work.

Supplemental Security Income (SSI) provides for a minimum income level for needy aged, blind and disabled
persons. Qualifications are determined by financial need
based on income and resources.

Individuals may qualify for only SSI benefits, only SSDI
benefits or both. Under both programs, eligibility is based
on mental or physical impairment expected to last at least a
year and preventing the person from being gainfully employed.

Vocational rehabilitation may provide additional benefits, including counseling, job guidance, training and placement. These services may be available whether or not the original disability claim is approved.

Medicaid benefits to help with health care costs are usually available to persons eligible to receive SSI.

Medicare benefits become available after one year on SSDI.

Social Security disability claims for narcolepsy must be filed under the impairment listing for Epilepsy. Although unusual, some claims have been approved as Organic Mental Disorders. Neither category, of course, is appropriate.

Because narcolepsy is considered a relatively rare disorder, it has never been given an impairment rating of its own. Consequently, claimants must battle a long line of obstacles and delays in order to be approved. It usually takes someone who "knows the ropes," such as an attorney who is familiar with Social Security cases, to follow the process through to a successful completion. For help in locating such an attorney, contact National Organization of Social Security Claimants' Representatives, 19 E. Central Avenue, Pearl River, N.Y. 10965; 1-800/431-2804.

The powers that have authority over these listings should take immediate action to correct this inequity. It is understandable that narcolepsy was given an inappropriate listing years ago, but it is inexcusable for this obstacle to remain in the path of handicapped persons.

The Developmentally Disabled Assistance and Bill of Rights Act is a federal statute providing federal funds to states for special programs. Information may be obtained from local developmental disability offices.

LEGISLATION PROHIBITING DISCRIMINATION

If you have been or are being discriminated against by your employer because of problems related to narcolepsy, you no longer have to suffer in silence. The following federal acts prohibit discrimination against persons with disabilities and provide for accommodations in the workplace.

The Rehabilitation Act of 1975 was the first comprehensive federal law to prohibit employment discrimination based on handicaps. It also provided rehabilitation and independent living programs for disabled persons unable to obtain, retain or prepare for employment. Further, it required employers under federal law to make reasonable allowances and adjustments to meet the needs of handicapped employees.

The Americans with Disabilities Act (ADA) of 1990 (Public Law 101-336, 1990, 42, U.S.C. S12101 et seq.) provides equal opportunities to qualified disabled individuals in the areas of employment, state and local government services, transportation and public accommodations.

You have the legal right to be accommodated, but your employer has the legal right to deny your request if it creates an undue hardship. If you and your employer cannot arrive at an acceptable agreement, assistance can be obtained from the EEOC, state or local rehabilitation agencies or from disability constituent organizations. For information, look in the government pages of your phone book under Equal Employment Opportunities Commission (EEOC), or contact:

Job Accommodation Network
918 Chestnut Ridge Road, Suite 1
West Virginia University
P.O. Box 6080
Morgantown, WV 26506-6080
   Job accommodation information: 1/800/526-7234
   ADA information: 1/800/232-9675

A service of the President's Committee on Employment of People With Disabilities, this international consulting service provides information about job accommodation and the employability of people with job disabilities.

Insurance Problems

People with narcolepsy quite frequently have problems with insurance. Some companies will not provide health insurance for anyone with narcolepsy. Others may grant coverage with a rider excluding narcolepsy. And some will cover narcolepsy as a pre-existing condition after a period of time. Yet others will provide immediate coverage if the applicant has not had any problems relating to narcolepsy within a given period of time. The companies that will write policies often raise their rates due to narcolepsy. If you are unable to get any insurance company to accept you, ask for information on high risk insurance pools. Of course, all of this will change—if and when we get national health care reform.

Some of these problems also pertain to life insurance. If you get life insurance, you will most likely be given a high risk rating with a higher premium.

Here are a couple of tips to use when applying for insurance:

□ Narcolepsy is a neurological, physical condition. Be sure it is not classified as a mental illness. Insurance companies typically pay a lower rate of reimbursement for mental illness than they do for a physical disease.

□ Before applying for insurance, send for a copy of your medical file. The Medical Information Bureau (MIB) is a data bank used by 750 insurance companies, who collect and share information when you apply for individual life, health or disability insurance. You may obtain a copy of your MIB report from Medical Information Bureau, P.O. Box 105, Essex Sta., Boston, MA 02112; phone 617/426-3660.

You may also request your medical records from your doctor. Sometimes the wording of a report can be critical in determining whether or not you will be approved for insurance. If it is obvious that negative wording will disqualify you for acceptance, you might ask the doctor to write a letter to the insurance company rather than sending a copy of your medical record. If the doctor understands the situation, he may be able to word his report honestly, and in such a way that it will be approved. There was one recently reported case in which a person, who had not had coverage for narcolepsy in twenty years, was approved with a prescription card!

DRIVING ISSUES

The slogan for drinking drivers could easily be paraphrased, "If you sleep, don't drive. If you drive, don't sleep." This must apply equally to all drivers. While people with narcolepsy are frequently identified as the sleepy people, they are only a small portion of those who are at risk of falling asleep behind the wheel.

This information is not in any way intended to provide an excuse for people with narcolepsy who are not responsible drivers to drive when they are sleepy. There is no acceptable excuse for anyone doing that. But when politicians are pressured into doing something about the increasing number of sleep-related accidents, people with narcolepsy who are easily identifiable as sleepy people, do not want to become scapegoats.

Bill Baird, a narcoleptic who is a past president of the now defunct American Narcolepsy Association, was recently interviewed in a *20/20* segment on television. John Stossel expressed some concern about Bill's ability to stay awake while driving, and Bill asked in return, "Do you ever get sleepy when you're driving?" John hesitated a moment and then had to admit that he did. Bill then explained the difference between a normal person who gets sleepy while driving and a person who has been diagnosed as having narcolepsy.

A normal person thinks he can control his sleep. (While this is not true, most people believe it is and act on what they believe.) Over-confident in his ability to stay awake, he continues to drive.

A person with narcolepsy, especially one who has been diagnosed and is knowledgeable about the disorder, is aware of his vulnerability to falling asleep and his limited ability to control it. With this awareness, a person with narcolepsy is more likely to pull off the road at the first indication of sleepiness. Individuals can learn to identify the feeling of sleepiness when it begins, and train themselves to pull off the road for a brief nap. In addition, they are aware of many coping techniques for staying awake, and go prepared to use them. All these things work together to help make responsible people with narcolepsy safer than average drivers.

A guide for physicians, *Narcolepsy: Care and Treatment*, co-authored by William P. Baird and William C. Dement, M.D., Ph.D., Director of the Stanford University Sleep Research Laboratory, states: "The accident rate of diagnosed patients with narcolepsy is lower than that of normal drivers." There are some people whose driving is not limited at all by their narcolepsy. There are others (like myself) who should not drive on the highway by themselves but can drive for short periods to relieve another driver. And yet others (like myself) who can drive in town. And then, there are those who should never drive.

Especially in matters of driving, we narcoleptics would do well to borrow from the Alcoholics Anonymous' serenity prayer which says, "God, grant me the serenity to accept the things I cannot change, the courage to change the things I can, and the wisdom to know the difference."

One major difference between diagnosed and undiagnosed narcoleptics is that those who have been identified are most likely taking medications. For many, stimulants make the difference as to whether or not they are able to drive. By proper timing of their medications to coordinate with their driving, plus the precautions mentioned above, people with narcolepsy can be among the best drivers on the road. Each one must be accountable to self, to passengers and to others on and off the road.

Hopefully, when the issue of removing "at risk" drivers comes up for consideration, legislators will find some fair and equitable way of solving this problem. Surely they can find some way that will not unjustly penalize responsible, safe drivers just because they have been diagnosed as having narcolepsy.

The laws regarding driver's licenses differ so greatly from state-to-state that no attempt will be made here to address the problem except to acknowledge it exists.

19
SOURCES OF INFORMATION AND ASSISTANCE

Center of Narcolepsy Research
University of Illinois at Chicago
845 South Damen Avenue (M/C 802)
Chicago, IL 60612-7350
312/996-5176; Fax 312/996-7008
Supervised by faculty and staff of UIL College of Nursing. Provides general information on narcolepsy, including referrals to state and federal resources, accredited sleep disorders centers and narcolepsy support groups. UIL at Chicago is a nonprofit educational organization; informational services of the Center must be fully funded by private donations.

Narcolepsy Institute
Montefiore Medical Center
111 East 210th St.
Bronx, NY 10467
212/920-6799
Information on narcolepsy, referrals; screening, case management, long and short-term counseling; in-service training and educational presentations; annual conference for patients and professionals. Their *Narcolepsy Primer: A Guide for Physicians, Patients and Their Families* is an excellent source of information. They are in the process of making a videotape about narcolepsy which will be available sometime in 1995.

Narcolepsy Network, Inc.
Box 1365, FDR Station
New York, NY 10150
914/834-2855
   The only currently existing national, nonprofit organization; founded and operated primarily by volunteers with narcolepsy. Provides general information on accredited sleep disorder centers and/or specialists, locating and forming support groups, filing disability or discrimination claims, etc. Provides list of free and inexpensive educational materials on narcolepsy upon request. Membership fee of $25 for individuals, $50–$100 for professionals/medical facilities; includes newsletter. Excellent *Guide To Understanding Narcolepsy* for new members. Annual conference each fall.

National Sleep Foundation
1367 Connecticut Ave. NW, Suite 200
Washington, DC 20036
202/785-2300
   Established by the American Sleep Disorders Association, the organization of professionals in sleep disorders medicine. Serves as a national referral service and coordinating center for public information; provides list of accredited sleep disorders centers; publishes a quarterly newsletter. No memberships; accepts contributions.

National Narcolepsy Helpline
415/591-7884
   Volunteer answers questions about narcolepsy; sends out general information and locations of sleep disorders centers and specialists.

20
REFERENCES

Aldrich, Michael S., MD. 1992. "Narcolepsy." *Neurology* 42 (SUPPL 6:34–43).

American Narcolepsy Association. *The Eye Opener* newsletters 1984–1993. San Francisco, CA.

Broughton, R. and Q. Ghanem. 1976. "The Impact of Compound Narcolepsy on the Life of the Patient." In C. Guillenminault, W.C. Dement and P. Passouant, eds. *Narcolepsy: Advances in Sleep Research*. New York: Spectrum, pp. 201–219.

Dement, William C., MD, PhD and Baird, William P. 1977. *Narcolepsy: Care and Treatment*.

Diagnostic Classification Steering Committee, Thorpy, M.J., Chairman. 1990. *International Classification of Sleep Disorders: Diagnostic and Coding Manual*. Rochester, MN: American Sleep Disorders Association.

Flapan, Mark, PhD. "Experiences of Living With a Rare Disorder." *NORD: Orphan Disease Update Supplements 1992–1993*.

Fleming, Jonathan A.E., Mb, FRCP(C) and Shapiro, Collin M., BSc(HON), MBBCh, PhD, MRC Psych., FRCP(C) 1992. *Sleep Solutions, Vol. 2: Insomnia Management*. Under the auspices of Sleep/Wake Disorders Canada. St-Laurent, Quebec: Kommunicom Publications.

Foulkes, David. 1966. *The Psychology of Sleep*. New York: Charles Scribner's Sons.

Fritz, Roger, PhD. 1993. *Sleep Disorders: America's Hidden Nightmare*. Grawn, MI: Publishers Distribution Service.

Fry, June M., MD, PhD. 1988. "Narcolepsy." *Encyclopedia Britannica, Inc.*

Goswami, Meeta, et al, eds. 1992. *Psychosocial Aspects of Narcolepsy.* Binghampton, NY: The Haworth Press, Inc.

Goswami, Meeta, MPH, PhD and Thorpy, Michael J., MD. 1991. *Narcolepsy Primer: A Guide for Physicians, Patients and Their Families.* Bronx, NY: Montefiore Medical Center.

Hanly, Patrick J. and Shapiro, Collin. 1992. *Sleep Solutions, Vol 4: Excessive Daytime Sleepiness.* Under the auspices of Sleep/Wake Disorders Canada. St-Laurent, Quebec: Kommunicom Publications.

Kryger, Meir H., MD, FRCPC; Roth, Thomas, PhD and Dement, William C., MD, PhD. 1994. *Principles and Practice of Sleep Medicine,* second edition. W.B. Saunders Company.

Luce, Gay Gaer and Segal, Julius. 1966. *Sleep.* New York: Lancer Books, Inc.

Mitler, Merrill M., PhD and Gujavarty, K.S., MD. "Narcolepsy: When to suspect it and how to help." *Consultant,* Jan. 1981, pp. 215–224.

Narcolepsy Network, Inc. 1994. *Narcolepsy: A Guide to Understanding.* New York.

Narcolepsy Network, Inc. *The Network* newsletters, 1986–1994.

Standards of Practice Committee of the American Sleep Disorders Association, Thorpy M.J., MD, Chairman. 1993. ASDA Consensus Statement.

APPENDICES

W HEN RESEARCH is conducted, all factors influencing the
outcome must be reported. If not, the study is considered flawed. That principle also holds true for my experiences. I *must* report all factors directly influencing my ability
to cope with narcolepsy.

It would have been inappropriate to mention my faith
in the main part of the book. People are of many diverse
religions, and this book is addressed to them all. Yet it is *my
Christian faith* that has helped me—beyond all else—to
successfully deal with my problems. It has a direct bearing
on all that I think and do and am. My faith is not an appendix
to my life, as it is to this book.

I could not fail to include this section, but you may choose
whether or not you want to read it.

NOTE: Any reviews or endorsements of this book do not
extend to the Appendices.

MY EVER-PRESENT HELP
IN TIME OF TROUBLE
(Ps. 46:4)

I AM GOING to devote a separate chapter to this testimony. You can skip over it and still have all the facts I have to offer about narcolepsy. But you cannot skip over it and understand how I cope.

Throughout my writing, I have related many stories of how I have successfully coped with specific problems. But I have not told you the *real* reason for *my* success and, unless I do, my book will be without integrity. I'll tell you now — His name is Jesus.

A few years ago, my husband and I attended an audio-visual class on relationships by Gary Smalley of Paoli, PA. In introducing the bonding process, whereby relationships are brought closer together and cemented, Gary said the best bonding often takes place on camping trips. He was quick to explain it is not the camping per se that acts as the cement, but the working together as a unit to meet the many emergencies that arise.

Bonding takes place, too, between the Lord and His children. The more troubles we have, the more opportunity there is for bonding. I must confess that I don't look forward to problems with that idea in mind. But I have had a lot of trauma and heartache in my life, and the Lord has been with me through it all. He never promised freedom from problems, sorrow, toil, pain and death. But the Lord did promise all who put their faith in Him, "I will never leave you nor forsake you" (Heb. 13:5).

My first big bonding experience came when I was twelve years old. Up until that time, my life was as near perfect as anything on this earth can be. My parents, who were teacher-administrators by profession, had been married thirteen years when I was born in 1934. I was an only child, and no child was ever more welcomed and more loved than I was. We were a wonderfully happy family, and I was a Daddy's girl.

In 1945, something happened to change that. Daddy developed the first symptoms of Alzheimer's Disease. His was the type that developed at an early age and progressed very rapidly. (Studies indicate there is a fifty per cent chance of offspring inheriting this form of the disease, but I won't worry because I am not a statistic with the Lord!) The last time I saw Daddy, while he could still talk, he said two things I'll never forget. He asked me, "Will you remember your daddy?" And he said, "Let's pray God's Will be done." Before I saw him the next time, he had lapsed into a vegetative state. He died about six weeks later. The faith of my earthly father left its mark upon my life—always pointing me toward my Heavenly Father. I have never doubted for a moment that his death was a part of God's Will.

Periodically, in connection with any tragedy, we hear the question, "Why did this happen?" Abruptly on the heels of this question, we often hear another, "How could a loving God allow this to happen?" Many times I have to accept by faith rather than have a specific answer to the first question. But I can accept whatever happens (including my narcolepsy) based on my knowledge of, and experience with, a loving God.

Sometimes our problems are clearly the consequences of our own wrong actions. If we eat too much fat and cholesterol, we are likely to develop heart problems. If we drive when we are sleepy, we are at risk of having an accident. God gave us the free will with which to make choices.

However, the choices we make often come with attached consequences.

But sometimes bad things happen to good people and that is a harder issue to deal with. For me, acceptance of unfavorable circumstances sometimes has to come via a process of working through what I know to be true. This involves the following questions, which I ask myself and answer:

- [ ] Does God love me and want His best for me at all times? *Yes*
- [ ] Does God know about this situation? *Yes*
- [ ] Does God care about this situation and its effect upon those involved, including me? *Yes*
- [ ] Can God do something about this problem—solve it, cure it, or change it? *Yes*

Since the answers to all the above are *yes* and the problem still exists, I must conclude that (a) God is allowing this to happen or (b) God is causing this to happen. It then follows that God is either allowing or causing this to happen *for some purpose*. For years I stopped here, but later added the following:

Since all God's purposes are good, I must accept by faith that this is happening for a *good* purpose. Regardless of the circumstances, this must always be my final conclusion. That settles it! God is in control and that is as it should be.

When I was seven years old, I received Jesus Christ as my Savior. Trusting God with my eternal life was a once-for-all commitment, but trusting God with my earthly life is an ongoing process. Each new problem that arises is a challenge to my faith and must be dealt with on an individual basis. Ultimately, I must decide whether or not I believe God when He said, "All things work together for good to them that love God,..." (Rom. 8:28).

In some cases, I will never know how God used that particular issue to bring about some good thing in my life.

If I am looking for material benefits, I may never see past the end of my nose. But God specializes in the spiritual realm—in spiritual blessings, closer bonding with Him and the peace of God that passes all understanding! Because I have experienced all these things, I can bear witness to God's marvelous grace.

My spiritual faith is not just something *extra* that helped me cope with narcolepsy. It gives meaning to my life and puts a song in my heart, whatever the circumstances.

Poem

When doubts and fears my fondest hopes assail,
    And dismal seems to be my destined lot;
My cry of woe becomes a tearful wail,
    And life itself but a dull, dreary plot.

I humbly kneel and look to God in prayer
    To search for solace in His holy face;
In His abiding love I am aware
    Of perfect peace and ever-saving grace.

How thankless then do I condemn myself
    For all the richest blessings heaped on me,
My cup runs over in spiritual wealth,
    No greater gift in life could ever be.

Let us ask not life's pleasures without pain,
    The sunshine is more welcome after rain.

by Marguerite Jones Utley

Written in 1965 in English Literature class at The University of Texas at Austin (a year prior to receiving a diagnosis of narcolepsy).

ADDRESS CORRECTIONS AND ADDITIONS

Narcolepsy Network, Inc.

E-mail: narnet@aol.com
http://www.websciences.org/narnet/

National Narcolepsy Registry (NNR)
Contact NSF Narcolepsy Coordinator
Stephanie Capalbo (202) 785-2300
E-mail: nat.sleep@haven.ios.com

American Sleep Apnea Association
2025 Pennsylvania Ave NW, Suite 905
Washington DC 20006
(202) 293-3650, e-mail: asaa@nicom.
http://www.nicom.com/~asaa

Restless Legs Syndrome Foundation
4410 19th St NW, Suite 201
Rochester MN 55901-6624
http://www.rls.org/RLSF.htm

American Sleep Disorders Association (ASDA)
6301 Bandel Road, Suite 101
Rochester MN 55901
(507) 287-6001
http://www.asda.org/staff.html

National Sleep Foundation (NSF)
729 15th St NW, 4th Flr
Washington DC 20005
http://www.sleepfoundation.org

SUGGESTED READING:

SNORING & SLEEP APNEA, 2nd ed.
By Ralph Pascualy, MD, & Sally Soest
Demos Vermande, pub.

SLEEP THIEF (for Restless Legs Syndrone)
by Virginia Wilson
Arthur S. Walters, MD, ed.
Galaxy Books, Inc., pub.,
Orange Park, FL